HELP YOURSELF
TO
ULTIMATE
HEALTH

HELP YOURSELF
TO
ULTIMATE
HEALTH

Know the Causes, Symptoms, and Solutions to Optimal Health

Abdel Jaleel Nuriddin, ND, PhD

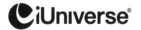

HELP YOURSELF TO ULTIMATE HEALTH
KNOW THE CAUSES, SYMPTOMS, AND SOLUTIONS TO OPTIMAL HEALTH

iUniverse books may be ordered through booksellers or by contacting:

iUniverse
1663 Liberty Drive
Bloomington, IN 47403
www.iuniverse.com
1-800-Authors (1-800-288-4677)

Because of the dynamic nature of the internet, any web addresses or links contained in this book may have changed since publication and may no longer be valid. The views expressed in this work are solely those of the author and do not necessarily reflect the views of the publisher, and the publisher hereby disclaims any responsibility for them.

Any people depicted in stock imagery provided by Getty Images are models, and such images are being used for illustrative purposes only. Certain stock imagery © Getty Images.

ISBN: 978-1-5320-4386-4 (sc)
ISBN: 978-1-5320-4387-1 (e)

Library of Congress Control Number: 2018902357

Print information available on the last page.

iUniverse rev. date: 03/27/2018

CONTENTS

REVIEWS

D<small>R</small>. A<small>BDEL</small> J. Nuriddin, ND, PhD, is one of the most prolific writers addressing the health and well-being of the individual from a holistic perspective. One of his strong points is his consistency in marrying what we eat to the outcome of our health.

Dr. Nuriddin's *Help Yourself to Ultimate Health* is a guidebook that breaks down in an easy-to-understand perspective why "sustained action" is necessary for longevity in good health. It cannot be hit-and-miss, but let it become a lifestyle with the purpose of good health. He intertwines the virtues of Al-Islam, where the individual's body has rights on him or her. Therefore, "preventive health care" is mandatory.

Of especial value is his ability/expertise/knowledge of how the body's early development gives clues to its maintenance—from the "primitive gut tube" to the woes of digestive deficiencies when certain enzymes are depleted to the cleansing of the blood/life source and then in maintenance mode on to the four seasons and what parts of the anatomy to attend to in their respective seasons.

He warns us to stop "drugging" ourselves when the body maintains its own abilities to cure itself—if given the right nutrients, including *water* with the proper pH balance. Rather than making drug companies billions in revenue, he says our pursuit of good health naturally will be its own economic reward without compromising our health or our integrity.

The Holy Qur'an tells us to "save yourselves and your family from hellfire" (66:6). Dr. Nuriddin demonstrates how our eating habits impact our health and how if we pass on proper knowledge to our children, we are indeed saving ourselves and our families from hellfire.

We thank Allah for Prophet Muhammed, through whom He revealed Al-Qur'an and then demonstrated the divine book via his very life as his wife Aesha said, "The Prophet was the Qur'an walking." In that spirit, Dr. Nuriddin has written a book that walks us through life's road to a healthy future, avoiding the pitfalls of bad habits and poor consumption that leads to a poor life—physically, mentally, and spiritually. He writes from a wealth of experience.

Thank you, Dr. Nuriddin, for sharing your twenty-plus years of knowledge—unselfishly—through the pages of the *Muslim Journal* weekly newspaper. And congratulations on the release of your new book, *Help Yourself to Ultimate Health*.

As-Salaam-Alaikum, the greeting that is a prayer for peace, obligating the one who gives it and the one who receives it to the peace of the Creator.

—Ayesha K. Mustafaa, editor, *Muslim Journal*

#

I am deeply honored and thankful to be asked to give a review of what I will call a must-read. I have had the pleasure of knowing Dr. Nuriddin over the past thirty years. In that period I have seen 100 percent of his dedication to health, wellness, and prosperity. I have been blessed to work with him over the years. We have joint ventures in marketing health and wellness products. He has been my health coach and spiritual leader throughout our prosperous relationship. Even as of this writing, after so many decades, we are still working together on bringing new category-creating, seed-based nutrition supplements to market. I am honored to say a few words regarding this incredible book.

I suggest you invest your valuable time, money, and energy in endeavors that are worthy. This book is an absolute treasure. Believe me—it is priceless. As you read it, you will discover the rewards of your investment. If you study one section in the book, it sums up the entire message. Developing the ability to do or taking the proper action—without being forced—is a great achievement in life. Having the vision and taking the next step, because you know or sense it's the proper thing to do, will always produce results.

I yield to the thoughts of Sir Isaac Newton's law of cause and effect. "For every action there is an equal and opposite reaction. Every human thought, word, and deed is a cause that sets off a wave of energy throughout the universe, which in turn, creates the effect—whether desirable or undesirable." This philosophy illustrates that in order for you to achieve *ultimate health, you must take action.*

The knowledge in this book will enhance your ability to take better control of your life, especially in health. You will acquire the simple knowledge of what is needed to focus on self-care versus health care.

Books can give complicated medical details that become so overwhelming that the layperson is inundated and frustrated. When this occurs, the reader is confused, so the message is lost. Dr. Nuriddin provides an opportunity to understand not only the medical information but the practical application as well. This is a refreshing approach to health and wellness. He offers personal anecdotes that relate strongly to the topic. You are taken on a journey of self-discovery while enjoying the ride.

It is no accident that this book is titled *Help Yourself to Ultimate Health*. When you go to a buffet, you *help yourself.* Therefore, *you* are an intricate element in achieving ultimate health. *Your* participation is required in reaching optimal wellness. Dr. Abdel Nuriddin takes you by the hand in this comprehensive maze and guides you safely to become a better you.

There are no books on the market that allow this glimpse into universal medical conditions through personal revelation. By the end of this book, you will relate to the author and his family. By the end of this book, you will understand what you need to do to improve your personal health concerns. By the end of this book, you will have a grasp of medical terminology that will assist you in everyday life. But most of all, by the end of this book, you will be empowered with knowledge that will uplift you to *help yourself to ultimate health.*

—Dr. Ali Yasin, doctorate of philosophy; founder and CEO of the Billionaire Mastermind Forum and Billionaire Mastermind University; author of *The Science of Thinking Rich*; and cancer survivor

#

Help Yourself to Ultimate Health is a very informative book that consists of many different topics. It gives a wider perception of how we should take precautionary measures on what's put in the body. The author helps us to understand how the human body cells perform, learning the different aspects of the body.

The book also contains information that will be beneficial to young mothers in understanding the eating habits of a child. For example, he speaks of how introducing a child to different types of food too soon can trigger food allergies, which play a substantial part in the child's intake. People who read this book will become knowledgeable on body development and function.

Dr. Nuriddin has written a book, and he is knowledgeable about the body wellness of people. It will *transform the way you learn about medicine* altogether. It is a guide to good health. He speaks to the readers in such a simplified way that even a child can understand. There is a lot of truth within the pages of this book. It has an excellent organizational setup and gives a lot of preventive information to a well-rounded, diverse group of people.

He speaks of not only our health but the cleanliness that our bodies need during certain parts of the year that will help prevent diseases. He helps us to understand the human body and how important it is to stay healthy. A brilliant author who knows the value of food and water and what they do for the body.

Reading this book has enlightened me in many ways. I would encourage you to get this book and take your time in reading each word written on each page. You can learn and understand preventative wellness, food, and cleanness, and we can understand more about a better human body development of a healthy life. It would help you to know more about how the body functions.

Dr. Nuriddin, thank you for a well-written book.

—Joyce Morant

#

Society is attempting to function in a dispensation where they place much emphasis on health and wellness. The medical profession spends large fortunes on drugs and physical therapy only to discover that individuals continue to be unhealthier than ever before. The traditional wellness profession recommends changes but continues to spend more time developing ways to make money than ways to correct the numerous health and wellness issues.

Dr. Nuriddin's approach concentrates on correcting body and mental functions. His concepts are based upon individual body metabolism and structure and not on what I call the "pill concept." Society designs a pill for every problem and then attempts to deal with the side effects later. Dr. Nuriddin addresses causes first and proper methods to correct the problem.

I highly respect these methods and recommend his concept.

—John Wesley M., DTh

DISCLAIMER

ABDEL JALEEL NURIDDIN, ND, PhD, is in no way involved in the diagnosis or treatment of disease. His diplomas and degrees have been earned and awarded by various institutions for his indulgence, research, and dedication to the physical, mental, and spiritual well-being of his fellow man in the fields of natural health and spiritual awakening.

A POEM

Body and mind and Spirit, all combine
To make the creature, human and Divine.
Of this great Trinity, no part deny.
Affirm, affirm, the great eternal I.
Affirm the body, beautiful and whole,
The earth-expression of immortal soul.
Affirm the mind, the messenger of the hour,
To speed between thee and the Source of power.
Affirm the Spirit, the eternal I—
Of this great Trinity, no part deny.

—Ella Wheeler Wilcox

FOREWORD

URING MY CAREER in clinical medicine, I have witnessed a paradigm shift in the field of health care. Today people are realizing the importance of the adage "An ounce of prevention is worth a pound of cure." Costly, high-tech, scientific medicine has had to admit that it is far more comfortable treating disease than it is promoting a low-cost, less glamorous health and wellness. For clinical medicine, health and wellness is like sailing into uncharted waters without the benefit of its tangible landmarks for disease processes. Moreover, medicine has finally conceded that health and wellness is much more than merely the absence of detectable disease. In fact, health and wellness represent the opposite end of the spectrum, which includes the wellspring of spiritual health.

With this understanding, it is my pleasure to introduce Dr. Abdel Nuriddin's timely, dynamic book. Dr. Nuriddin's origins are centered in the health and wellness end of the health spectrum, and from that position he discusses spiritual health, wellness, and disease treatment. This book represents a natural evolution and correction of a much earlier book with roots in health promotion and disease prevention. That book is *How to Eat to Live* by the late Honorable Elijah Muhammad. Dr. Nuriddin's book acknowledges the spiritual transformation that has occurred from the former Nation of Islam to the universal faith of Al-Islam under Imam W. Deen Mohammed, the son of the Honorable Elijah Muhammad.

Standard clinical medicine has been slow to recognize that indeed other health practitioners oftentimes come from clinical traditions that were time-tested over thousands of years. These health practitioners have been successfully treating many medical conditions long before the development of Western scientific medicine, and they have also been treating them at a fraction of the cost of Western medicine today. This fact—as well as the popular demand for alternative medicine throughout the world today—has forced Western medicine to move over and make room at the health care table for other health practitioners and new points of view.

Clinical scientific medicine has nearly come full circle and returned to its origins. Perhaps one day it may even recognize that God is the source of all healing.

—Mikal Ramadan, MD

INTRODUCTION

ABDEL NURIDDIN WAS born in Buffalo, New York, on June 13, 1946. His father was not in the household, and his mother was poor. With three brothers and three sisters, he pretty much ate whatever was put on the table for consumption. Neither his mother nor his father had any background in health or nutrition. Abdel was raised a Baptist in the Christian church. He credits his spiritual foundation to those early days in Sunday school and singing in the choir. In those early days while living with his grandmother, he and his siblings had to go to church each Sunday. Abdel is a veteran of the Vietnam era. In 1972, when his life was without guidance, he joined the Nation of Islam under the leadership and guidance of the Honorable Elijah Muhammad, and shortly thereafter, he met his wife, Connie. He joined because he saw the discipline in the followers of that movement. While practicing the tenants of that movement, he started to learn about health and developed better eating habits. In his midtwenties, he developed a desire to work as a businessman and wear suits. In 1986, he met Ali Yasin in New York City at Malcomb Shabazz Mosque, and this shaped his focus on residual income. In 1986, Abdel and Connie, his wife of forty-two years, met Bill and Mildred Horosh. Bill was an iridologist and naturopathic doctor, and Mildred was a colon therapist and nutritional consultant. From Bill and Millie, he learned about iridology; tissue cleaning; and how to use herbs, vitamins, and minerals to create protocols for clients to build better health in mind and body. Since the early 1970s, Abdel's main interest has been awaking people to their ultimate human potential and excellent health. He shares his time with people throughout the globe, teaching and coaching on holistic health and creating protocols for his client base. Abdel believes the world is a great place to live in, and he would love to see more people healthy, happy, prosperous, and rich.

The accomplished naturopath and imam is married with three children. Imam Nuriddin established his faith in the religion of Al-Islam as a result of studying the Holy Qur'an, the Bible, and the life of Prophet Muhammed under the adeptness of Imam W. Deen Mohammed. Preceding that research was his initial practice of Islam in 1972 under the leadership of the Honorable Elijah Muhammad. He received his BA and MA in nutrition in 1993 from the American Holistic College of Nutrition in Birmingham, Alabama. Dr. Nuriddin also earned a PhD in holistic nutrition from the American Holistic College of Nutrition. His doctorate degree in naturopathy is from the Clayton School of Natural Healing, which is also in Birmingham, Alabama. Dr. Nuriddin has studied with Dr. Bill Horosh, Dr. E. C. Watkins, Mr. Michael Coyle, Dr. David Pesek, and Mr. John Andrews, master herbalist and iridologist of the United Kingdom. He is a diplomat of holistic iridology, a title he received from the International Institute of Iridology in 2008.

Today Dr. Nuriddin lives in Greensboro, North Carolina, where he owns and operates Genesis Health and Nutrition Center, LLC, with his wife, Connie. Dr. Nuriddin is also the author of *Causes, Symptoms, and Solutions* and coauthor of *The Five Essentials of Balanced Health*.

The great shift in consciousness from curative health care to preventive health care is touching every household in America today, just as the new trends of rap and hip-hop did. However, preventive health care is an old-world *trend* that's being renewed for some people and birthed for others in North America. This new trend of preventive health care will stay with the American public until the Creator Himself changes the universal order of things because it is and has always been in alignment with the nature of all humankind.

The curative side of health care (or allopathic medicine), which primarily focuses its attention on medication, sedation, and invasive operations, is very questionable today in the mind of the contemporary public relative to its effectiveness in cure. Drugs and pharmaceuticals that at one time in America's history were a panacea for our health care are today seen and known as something with latent and harmful side effects. While this form of medicine is doing much to save the lives of many humans throughout the globe, its lack of emphasis on prevention and more effective treatment is now shadowing its great advancements. While America is great in its technological advancements, it is also great in its sickness. We cannot blame this all on allopathic medicine, but what allopathic medicine does have to take responsibility for are the consistent negative side effects of each drug and the daily operations that medical professionals say are senseless and unnecessary. The lack of education about illness and people not taking responsibility for their own health is equally as negative.

Because of many great thinkers in this new age, including Dr. Bernard Jensen, Victor E. Irons, Dr. Bill Horosh, and others, more Americans are going back to nature in terms of health care. The importance of internal organ cleansing and the utilization of herbs and enzymes are techniques that are once again finding their way into the mind of the public. This is the course to follow to get out of the dark corridors of America's health care system. *Help Yourself to Optimal Health* is a book of papers and essays devoted to shining a light on a dark street that needs illumination to help preserve the public's health. I thank Allah, my wife, Connie, my family, and the many teachers and mentors who have had a hand in shaping my mind. Their influence has led to the publication of this material, which is designed to improve the health of the reader. May Allah's grace and mercy be upon you all.

A BIT ABOUT WATER AND TODAY

THE WORLD OF atoms (electrons, protons, and neutrons) has the energy of the original substance running through them, and this is what gives the elements life. Whether we're talking about minerals that are inanimate, plant life with its restricted movement, or animal and human life with emotion and intelligence, it all comes from the same substance and common origin. While this common substance (water) that all living matter comes from has the constituents of two atoms of hydrogen and one atom of oxygen, the elements are not always in that order in certain molecules. This means that while hydrogen and oxygen can be in the same matter, the matter does not have to be in liquid form. For instance, all paper has the constituents of water in it, which makes it flexible, but it's not liquid. However, if the elements were not there, the paper would not bend. The less hydrogen and oxygen, the less flexible a thing is.

The Holy Qur'an states that every living thing comes from water and must have water to exist (21:30). If we think about this substance or these particles that originate from the universal substance or source energy, then we realize they must be pure in their natural state. Maybe that is why all babies are so flexible and clean.

The more water we have in our bodies, the more flexible or alive our bodies are. The less water, the stiffer or more lifeless our bodies are. When all the moisture leaves the body, rigor mortis sets in. Water cannot be underutilized in healthy living.

The reference to man's evolution on this planet would cause us to agree that there are grades of water ranging from pure to toxic. This tells us that all water is not equal in quality. Hence, the quality of life in the body is affected by the quality of the water consumed. The body is composed of

75 percent water. This means that water is the biggest element in the body, which stands to reason that you need more water each day than all the other elements combined. The proper ratio of water consumption daily for the human body varies depending on who you are talking to. Some say we should drink eight eight-ounce glasses per day. Others say that drinking when you are thirsty is adequate. I subscribe to the view that it is best to drink half of your weight in ounces daily to prevent sickness stemming from dehydration. This could vary with chronic kidney disease. If you are thirsty, the internal organs are already dehydrated. The water in each body must be clean to ensure good health. Dr. David Carpenter presents a good analogy when he talks of fish in the fishbowl. The fish are suspended in water that has a certain purity. The pH (potential for the expression of hydrogen) is also a part of this equation of purity. As we maintain a certain pH in the bowl, the fish stay healthy. However, if you fail to keep the water pH balanced (in an alkaline state), the fish will die. Our cells are suspended in blood (fluids) just as the fish are. The proper pH for the blood is 7.365 to 7.4. The brain will negatively affect metabolism to keep the blood in the correct range for life. The brain instinctively knows when the blood is too acidic, and moves first to protect its own existence.

Why would the brain damage the body only to stop a more immediate death. When the bloodstream becomes too acidic, then the brain starts making decisions that are in the best interest of the longevity of the whole body and not just a part. The bad acids must be controlled. Potassium, calcium, magnesium, among others are agents that buffer or control these acids. However, too many bad acids will drive these buffering agents out of the bloodstream. As an example, when this happens, the brain will begin to pull calcium out of the bones and teeth to buffer the acids. This leads to osteoporosis or bone and teeth disorders. Fluid pH should be a major component in your decision about water consumption and quality.

If the bad acid load on the body is too heavy, then it will cause the disintegration of tissue and create an environment where parasites and micro biotic life will thrive. The good news is that those lower forms of life don't like an alkaline bloodstream in the host.

Lastly, potassium, calcium, magnesium, and bicarbonates are already in your tap water in most cases. If you could get those buffering agents in your drinking and cooking water every day without getting the contaminants, that would be a real blessing in today's world. However, the chlorine, fluoride, rust, lime, and other chemicals in tap water—not to mention the parasites—must be filtered out, and are in some cases known carcinogens. Owning an ionizer helps to alkalize and gives you a clean drinking water. Visit www.alkaviva.com/drnuriddin for more information.

SUSTAINED ACTION IS NEEDED FOR GREAT RULES

WITHIN THIS BOOK you can find information about preventive health care. In addition, there is instruction for the practical application of this information. Knowledge alone is not enough to produce results. And results are the name of the game. Correcting our thinking, ceasing the intake of matter that causes disease, detoxing the body of what is contributing to the current problem, and then replenishing the body with the nutrients lost can and will produce favorable results. Also, getting plenty of rest, exercising regularly, keeping conscious of the divine intelligence, and subjecting oneself to vitreous meditation can help you in balancing your entire life.

Many people come up short in life because they fail to act in the appropriate way relative to what their objectives are. Developing the ability to take the proper action without being forced is a great achievement in life. Having the vision and taking the next step because you know it's the proper thing to do will always produce a result. In some cases, it is better to do something instead of nothing when faced with a decision that you do not know the outcome. We must be risk-takers in life. We must develop faith and learn how to make proper decisions and then evaluate our progress.

The psychologist tells us today that it's not that the human being cannot reach his or her goals, but rather the problem is that most don't know what they want or they don't set goals. One must learn how to focus on a specific objective until one reaches closure or gets results, *irrespective to how long it takes*. Achievement of any task first begins with the belief that one can achieve the task. Our Creator has given humans the potential for adaptability so that they can become what they need to be at any given time. This means they can accomplish any task that they put their minds to. After one believes he or she can achieve a goal, then one must take the initiative. Once action has been taken, one must evaluate the results. The evaluation of results is necessary to see if the action is moving one toward the desired outcome. You don't want to mistake movement for achievement. You could be acting, but not getting any closer to the objective. After you evaluate the current results, if they are not in accord with the desired objective, you must have the intelligence, the will, and the courage to change what or how you are doing what you're doing to offset any undesirable outcome.

To prevent yourself from making the same mistakes, you must learn to record the results. Also, recording results is the only way you can be sure that the next person can duplicate your progress without the same complications.

Putting systems in place develops institutions and helps remove chaos. The human body is made up of systems. It is the natural pattern that the Creator put in the human body as a sign of human social life. When the systems in the human body are not balanced, you will suffer from a disorder or disease in the body. To ensure the life of any organism, Allah gave it a system of functions, and that system supports the maintenance of the entire organism. The first complete system that Allah created was the atom. Then He created the cell and tissue and the organ. Organs make up greater systems, and these systems make up the entire body. Without this infrastructure and hierarchy, you cannot have biological life. And if some organs are missing from the body, you cannot have the healthiest life possible. Think health and consistent action and you will get the results you need.

PREVENTIVE HEALTH CARE: A DOMINANT THEME OF AL-ISLAM AND ALL RELIGIONS

IMAM W. DEEN Mohammed suggested in his transformation of the Nation of Islam, the keeping of the good practices of sensible behavior of his father's teaching in care of self. While the diet and eating habits of the Honorable Elijah Muhammad's followers carried on the surface obvious health benefits, beneath the surface there was an enticement for conscious evolution and change.

As the world finds itself in the new millennium, the need for renewed conscious concern in health habits face Muslims and other faith groups in America and throughout the world. These health habits must agree with the universal law for them to produce results on a broad scale. Peace of mind cannot be gained from prayer alone. It must work in conjunction with intelligent principles of consumption, internal cleansing, the will to work the body vigorously at times, and also adequate rest for the body and mind.

Allah says in the Qur'an (25:54), "And it is He who created man from water." Today science tells us that the human body is made up of 75 to 83 percent water. The brain, which controls every system in the human organism, is comprised of 83 percent water. If the human doesn't put adequate amounts of water into the body, then all systems will suffer from dehydration, and this is one of the leading causes of disease in humans. Water has as much importance today in our lives as it did at the inception of humankind's creation. The need for a minimum of six to eight eight-ounce glasses of water per day is just as crucial in this contemporary time as it was during the time of Adam, the first man. Water is a universal element that by itself cannot sustain life, but without it, you cannot have life. The proper amount of water is imperative for humans to lead healthy lives.

In the Qur'an (40:67), the Creator says, "It is he who created you from Turab or soil." In the soil are all the natural biological elements that make up the human body. The human body is produced out of the earth like a plant. The only difference comes in the process of reproduction. Plants are asexual, and humans are sexual. The human body manufactures sperm and ovum as a result of what it consumes. These cells, sperm, and ovum by themselves are incomplete, but when the sperm impregnates the ovum, the process of reproduction begins. After a period of gestation in the female womb, the completed form comes into the light of the sun (birth). In the sperm and ovum are water, minerals, phosphates, fats, carbohydrates, proteins and nucleic acids. These constituents must be in our diets regularly in the proper amounts for our bodies and minds to work in a healthy way. If there is an imbalance in these components, the human being will suffer disease. For example, too much sugar and simple carbohydrates can lead to diabetes. Too many saturated fats can lead to coronary heart disease. A deficiency in nucleic acids can lead to birth defects.

The Holy Qur'an (30:30) states that infinite intelligence says that He has created you on a pattern of Fitra (dynamism). In our universe dynamic activity leads to dynamic rest and vice versa. Under normal circumstances, the deeper we sleep the more exertion the body can stand, and the more exertion we give the body, the deeper we sleep. Allah says that He has created the day for livelihood (exertion) and that He has created the night for sleep (rest). This rest is necessary to rejuvenate the mind and body, and as a result, this gives our spirit a climate for its greatest expression—the worship of Allah or the acknowledgement of truth.

The greatest expression of the Creator's will is through the intellect of the human mind. The human's reason, and logic are the primary factors that separate the person from the animal kingdom. In the person's thinking processes, there are potential vibrations that lead to the health or sickness of the human body. In his publication "Keys to Success," Napoleon Hill says, "The expression of anger carries with it a vibration that can foster an arthritic (an inflamed) condition in the body. The expression of envy and jealousy carry with them the vibrations that can foster deficiencies of essential elements in the human body." These thoughts are restrictive to proper cell function and literally burn or drive vital nutrients out of the system, leaving the body bare and vulnerable to disease. The Qur'an and the traditions of our prophet Muhammed (PBUH) clearly suggest and state that we should eliminate the expression of anger and negative emotion. To the contrary, thoughts of peace, love, joy, happiness, moderation, and laughter are liberating for the human body. They open the cellular structure to proper excretion, secretion, digestion, and elimination and health.

The object of life is peace, and the acquisition of it comes through peaceful and balanced thinking. Regardless of ethnicity, color, nationality, gender, or religion, the Creator wants the same thing for all human beings in their ultimate expression, and that is peace.

Most humans have been taught all their lives that thought cleanliness is next to godliness. This is also true on a biological level. Cleanliness is next to healthiness. No longer can the earth's people only pay attention to cleaning the outside of their bodies and neglect their internal organs and expect to have good health. Sickness has become too great for people today to be ignorant of this natural fact. Among other things, we should subject ourselves—and suggest to our families—the health standard of internal cleansing each year. Your instinctive biological nature suggests you cleanse your filtering system (liver) in the springtime, that you cleanse your circulatory system (cardio care) in the summer, that you cleanse your respiratory system (lungs and bronchioles) in the fall, and that you cleanse the mineral- and electrolyte-balancing system (kidneys) in the winter. At least once per quarter, we should cleanse the bowel (colon). Developing and practicing this conscious healthy behavior will ultimately lead to a lifestyle that will support preventive health care as the dominant theme in our lives. Actually, this leads one to accord with true religion which suggest prevention and not cure as its uppermost theme.

Imam W. Deen Mohammed's commentary (Tafsir) on the Qur'an and the life of our prophet Muhammed (PBUH) has opened the way for a greater expression of human technology. The knowledge he has shared with his associates and other people today is influencing how the world's people will think about life in the future. Irrespective of what vocation you may bring to the table in regards to reason related to religion, health, economics, education, politics, and other professions, under the careful scrutiny of Imam Mohammed's teachings, your insight will become deeper.

WE MUST ALL THANK THE HONORABLE ELIJAH MUHAMMAD

W E MUST ALL thank the Honorable Elijah Muhammad for his great guidance, particularly in terms of self-care. I cannot forget his insistence that we eat to live. I, too, believe as he did that you see the world through the eyes of your stomach, metaphorically speaking. Food has a great effect on the body, mind, and spirit. And some food is really garbage, and it affects your ability to see clearly. He sought to keep his followers away from too much food and the wrong types of food, and those of us who followed him and obeyed his guidance returned from the sickness and spiritual death of poor eating habits. Most of his followers found him when they were sick from parasites from pork, white sugar, table salt, milk, white bread, white flour products, alcohol, and drugs. I will never forget, and I will never let my children forget, the Honorable Elijah Muhammad and his program, which gave life to so many people in and outside of the Nation of Islam.

I never met the man personally. When I encountered the Honorable Elijah Muhammad's program, I knew nothing about wellness or preventive health care. However, I was intrigued with the discipline that his followers had, much of which I realized later came from the discipline related to their dietary habits. One reason why the world didn't control his followers was because they had control of their stomachs. If you believe this is a lie, then I urge you to try to prove me wrong. Our attitudes were under better control because our personal spirit was better, and it was better because the temple (body) was cleaner and stronger. The Honorable Elijah Muhammad kept us away from as many acid-building foods, some of which were laced with cyanide, as he possibly could. Pork, white sugar, table salt, cow's milk, white bread, white rice, white flour products, alcohol, and drugs were not a part of his food regimen. If we are honest with ourselves, we must admit that these foods are just as poisonous today as they were during his time.

During his time the world outside the Nation of Islam, especially the United States, was experiencing more and more sickness because of fast foods, fillers, dyes, steroids, and hormones, to name a few. Elijah Muhammad's followers were enjoying vibrant health. Even our seniors were youthful in their appearance. After the loss of the Honorable Elijah Muhammad, no one told the followers of Imam W. Deen Mohammed to change their diets. They had freedom, and so they changed on our own volition. Imam W. Deen Mohammed emphasized and encouraged additional education that stimulated me and many others to specialize in various fields for the sake of community growth. We have acquired this knowledge in wellness and preventive health care for our entire community, and we have too much for just our immediate families. Allah wants us to live and live abundantly. Why should his followers throw away all the good that his father gave us and expect to progress in future generations? We must salvage the good. Only the foolish cast aside the good of the preceding generation and start all over again.

Dear people, if we don't get control of our stomachs, history will show Americans to be a foolish people after what they have been taught by the Honorable Elijah Muhammad. Was there more we needed to know beyond what he has taught us about health care? Yes, and others along with myself in this community today are in the process of teaching this information to America and the world.

AMERICAN'S NEED FOR ALTERNATIVE HEALTH CARE PRACTITIONERS

R ELIGION FOCUSES ATTENTION on every aspect of the human life. Despite what one may think under the influence of spiritualism, the physiological and biological aspects of a worshipper cannot be neglected, and the person must have total compliance with his or her religion.

Imam W. Deen Mohammed's association of Muslims in America and throughout the world is composed of a growing body of conscious adherents dedicated to the establishment of a total way of life that encompasses all that is good. This is for Muslims and non-Muslims alike, for this generation and all generations to come.

I believe that the perspective his followers have and the approach that they take as religious practitioners relative to health care today will influence in some way every generation to come in the religious community. I believe it is extremely necessary for all people of faith irrespective of their religion to have some knowledge of the curative side of health care. This is because most people today have some type of major or minor disorder. For some, these disorders come from innocent ignorance, and for other, they come from conscious neglect. Today many people are beginning to realize that they must take better care of their bodies. In addition, many people are realizing that if they die today before they reproduce, their community will be at a tremendous loss, whether they are Christian, Muslim, Jew, or other. However, I personally believe that it is even more important for as many of them as possible to learn about the preventive side of health care for the sake of future generations.

My sense is that all religions have a dominant theme of prevention instead of one involving cures. In the Holy Qur'an, Allah says to the

Muslim, "Save yourself and your family from a fire whose fuel is men and stones." This suggests to me that one must do something to prevent the inevitable misfortune if one engages or persists in improper conduct.

The history of every era of Al-Islam's evolution since our Prophet Muhammed (PBUH) has shown that the people of that time always produced from their own loins (community) or they attracted the professionals from Christians, Jews, and others in every field of life to perpetuate the Islamic community development, and the Muslims of this era must do the same in this contemporary movement. My primary focus in this book is on preventive health care (medicine), but this is true in every aspect of community building. Today our community needs more writers to preserve Imam Mohammed's *tafsir* (clear contemporary commentary on scripture). I believe our community's school of thought is centered on the preventive aspect of health care instead of the curative side. And if it is not, we will have serious problems in the future trying to preserve our contemporary mode of thinking. If you don't write (and publish) to preserve knowledge, when the Creator takes the body, He will also take the knowledge. Paraphrasing the Qur'an, Allah says, "If you will not accept the responsibility I have placed upon you, I will take it from you and give it to another people." I believe that the people who have been chosen today must publish to carry out the responsibility of passing that knowledge on, or they will lose the flavor that's in the responsibility. Ultimately, posterity becomes the greatest loser.

I am with Imam W. Deen Mohammed, helping with the mission that I believe Allah has placed upon him. I believe a great part of that mission is the dispensation of quality knowledge that gives humankind a better chance of living in accord with the will and the nature of our Creator, which ultimately preserves and stimulates the growth of human life. While I believe that most humans do the best they can with the resources they have, we can probably all stretch a little more if we attempted to improve our health, thereby setting the proper example for the next generation.

DEVELOPING A HEALTH CONSCIOUSNESS IS YOUR CREATOR'S WILL

AFTER ALMOST FIVE decades of developing particular habits, I am convinced that one must have a consciousness for health to attain it. When I say consciousness for health, I mean a dominant method of thinking about personal habits ranging from what one eats to how much rest you give yourself to how much exercise you are willing to do to maintain or regain your health.

As I understand the theme of the Holy Bible and the Holy Qur'an, these books of divine revelation suggest that humans should be aware of balance in all their affairs. And if we make an error or a mistake, then let it be in usefulness instead of selfishness. In the Holy Bible, Leviticus 19:35–36 (KJV) states, "Ye shall do no unrighteousness in judgment, in mete-yard, in weight, or in measure. Just balances, just weights, a just ephah, and a just hin, shall ye have." The Qur'an has many reference points alluding to this as well, including 55:7–9, which says, "Don't fall short in the balance ... Don't let your own hands contribute to your destruction ... Appetites should be checked by knowledge." The Qur'an also states that Al-Islam is the "midway religion," suggesting that those of us who practice it should be balanced in our personal habits.

How does one develop this health consciousness? First you must be aware that your Creator wants you to have it. Health consciousness is connected to the regard of the infinite intelligence. Instinctively, we as humans know that our bodies should be coordinated with our minds and shouldn't be in conflict with each other. In addition to first being aware of the Almighty's intention for you, the reading of health-conscious material, watching videos, listening to audiobooks, and attending and making available workshops and seminars on health will help in developing this health consciousness for yourself and others.

Should I eat out at fast-food chains? It's not recommended, but with today's lifestyle, most people will. Some of their food is not halal or kosher for Muslims. So in that vein, you must make a conscious religious decision. However, we should be mindful of the fact that the food of certain people (Christians and Jews) is lawful for Muslims. In regards to the content and the preparation of fast foods (saturated fat, heavy salt, sugar, and deep fried items), I would not recommend frequent consumption if possible. For us, the home cooking of our wives and mothers should in most cases be better for us than eating out. We should love and cherish our women cooking for us. The Muslim woman who is health conscious is a blessing to her immediate family and the community.

Today's world requires us to be more vigilant about our health. We must always ask, "Is this overdoing it?"

Monitor your consumption of foods, especially the ones that you know are unhealthy, because we all at times fall victim to our taste buds. Some of the most dangerous food today include too much sugar, white flour products, caffeine, salt, hormones and steroids in meat products, pasteurized and homogenized dairy products, fillers, dyes, preservatives, saturated fat, alcohol, and drugs, whether legal or illegal.

We must believe as Muslims that the first way of the Supreme Being is prevention and then cure, and having a strong regard for His presence relevant to your health will give you a health conscious mind and awareness.

BUILD YOUR FUTURE HEALTH NOW!

C AN PEOPLE BE certain that they will be in good health tomorrow? No, they can't. As believers in the Creator, we are encouraged to say, "If it is the will of Allah," when it comes to future events. Divine providence is in the power of your Lord, or we exist within the scheme of Allah's plan. It is the Creator who has taught people the natural law that governs the physical, mental, and spiritual worlds. While we cannot be totally certain about the future, educated people in most cases always fare better than the ignorant in planning for the future because of their knowledge of natural law, whether they recognize it as that or not. Allah has given people the ability to make strategies for future events if people know what they want. What better way to commence the rest of your life than learning how to develop and plan health strategies for you and your family?

As the first premise, you believe that your Creator wants you to be healthy, irrespective of what your health condition may be at present. Second, you must believe you are supposed to have good health, and third, you are to believe that you can and will have good health.

Next, we must know what good health is. My definition of good health is when the person has a balance (homeostasis) in and between body, mind, and spirit. Having balance in your body is when organs and systems are working together for the common good of the entire body. This can only happen when the cells that make up these organs and systems are nurtured with the proper nutrients, free of toxic waste, rested, exercised, and protected from harmful external pollutants. Having balance in your mind is when you are emotionally stable and your thinking is accurate. Spiritual stability is when a person accepts the Creator as the supreme authority in his or her life and seeks to understand Him and obey His laws.

Total health is harmony (balance) of body, mind, and spirit. It's when all these aspects of the person are working together for balance (health) in the entire organism.

The way in which Allah has created the human cell is nothing short of miraculous. The cell is made up of atoms, and cells make up tissues. There are too many different functions that the cell performs to discuss in this one essay. However, you should know the human cell has attached to it the possibility of homeostasis, hypo and hyper activity, the possibility of sickness or health, and the expectation of life and death.

When the cell has homeostasis it digests, assimilates, secretes, excretes, and eliminates based on the natural speed that the Creator assigned it. These functions make up what we call metabolism.

The direction of the cell at any given time is aimed toward sickness or health. In five years from now, you will either be healthier or sicker based on the direction of the cell today. Your sickness or health is influenced by your personal habits, which determine the direction of the cell. Your habits of eating and drinking, resting, exercising, thinking, worshipping, and cleansing all contribute to tomorrow's health or lack of it.

The life expectancy of the cell has to do with present habits of practice. The elements in the previous paragraph outline these habits. One's diagnosis today of eminent death in six months can change based on a change of habits today. Habits lead to pathology, and present pathology can be changed by developing new habits, which will ultimately change the duration or life expectancy of the cell diagnosed.

Since so many Americans are dying from cardiovascular disorders, such as heart attacks, strokes, high blood pressure, aneurysms, and other related maladies, let's examine why this is the case and look for some answers to offset these life extinguishers. If we were to look at our bodies from the perspective of being one single cell with various tissues serving diverse functions, perhaps we could understand better how to treat ourselves. As a cell, you came out of the earth like all other cells. Your biological mother and father ate the nutrients (food) from the earth, and they manufactured sperm and ovum in their bodies. After their sexual interaction, you were given life. You have the same composition of the matter (material) that makes up the earth. Water, fibers, gums, carbohydrates, proteins, fats, minerals, nucleic acids, and phosphates all make up the earth and your cell in this example. You need these things in balance for your metabolic processes to work properly. As a cell, you must produce heat and energy, secrete hormones, excrete fluids, eliminate waste, regulate body rhythms, control reproduction cycles, and the list goes on. Why isn't this happening in a healthy way for most cells in the cardiovascular system of people who live in America? Studies are showing that most American's lack adequate dietary fiber, magnesium, and lipase in their diets, and these deficiencies are major factors related to cardiovascular disorders.

What is the alternative? For instance, as a cell, you need at least fifteen to twenty grams of good dietary fiber each day beyond the nine to thirteen grams you are presently getting if you want to offset cardiovascular problems. If you have the problem already, you need to increase the intake of dietary fiber to improve your condition and decrease the chance of further complications.

We live in a time when more people between the ages of thirty to sixty are looking at preventive health care than ever in the history of this country. It would be encouraging if there is a decline of coronary heart disease among God-fearing people in this country, but there isn't. That is why I have written these essays, and I pray to the Lord they are hitting home. Personally, I have witnessed too many positive health results in people on a small level to believe we can't solve many of our health problems on a larger scale. We have to believe and take the necessary action for proper results. Now is the time to build your future health.

PROSTATE PROBLEMS

ONE OF THE most plaguing problems facing the American male today is the problem with his prostate. Statistics from the government sources state that four out of five men will have some type of prostate disorder by age sixty.

Today I don't have a prostate problem; however, because I fall within the problem age range, I see it necessary and crucial to consume daily herbal remedies, including saw palmetto, beta sitosterol, and stinging nettle, and to also examine all-natural health modalities to offset this disorder occurring in men between the ages of thirty-five and sixty. You can call my office and order Prostate Gold for supplementation. Men may also want to see a neurologist for the problem. When a member of the American family is plagued with prostate problems, it can cause extreme stress, leading to anxiety, depression, separation, and divorce.

In addition to the male being unable to perform his manly duties with his spouse, the cost of treatment also takes its toll on the family. However, even though most men today don't know the cause of the problem, many are becoming aware of preventive and curative methods to address the issue.

The twentieth century was probably the most exciting and progressive time in the history of humankind's earthly evolution. Industrialization, automation, communication, aviation, cyberspace, radio, and television have propelled the human species into modern times. However, it is a dangerous time in terms of the individual's personal health as people proceed toward their personal destiny. The development of pasteurization, homogenization, steroids, and artificial hormones, among other chemicals, has taken its toll on the public. Excessive alcohol consumption, tobacco smoking, taking illegal and legal drugs, fast-food eating, and environmental pollutants are all contributing factors to the ill health of our public. If the American government and private foundations don't incorporate preventive health care into public sphere, then future generations will be even sicker than we are.

The prostate is a gland in the male mammal composed of muscular and glandular tissue that surrounds the urethra at the bladder. It is called the prostate gland, and it serves as a sex accessory gland.

Protecting the prostate in light of today's harmful diet and environmental factors is becoming a must for the American male. Developing an awareness of the prostate and the function it serves is one of the most important steps in protecting the gland. Being aware of the problems associated with the prostate gland could alleviate personal disorders and grief. But since most men don't know they have a prostate until a problem arises, this task must somehow in part become a responsibility of those in society who do know about these issues.

While many men are becoming aware of prostate problems because someone they know had or is experiencing some disorder, there is not enough mass education on the problem to bring the statistics down. In the United States, there has been a 30 percent increase of men being diagnosed with prostate cancer each year. In 1995, 244,000 American men were diagnosed with prostate cancer, and in 1996, 317,000 were diagnosed with the disease. Statistics say one in nine men who are fifty years or older is diagnosed with prostate cancer each year. Organizations such as the Center for Disease Control (CDC) point out that African American men have an even higher rate of prostate cancer. The lack of early detection, the consumption of foods high in fat, and the lack of resources for medical exams have been cited for the higher rates among the African American males. The CDC also states that prostate cancer is the second most common form of cancer among American men (next to colon cancer).

I hope that those men reading this chapter will have themselves checked for this problem, if they are experiencing frequent urination, dribbling after urination, a lack of erection, pain in the lower back, and a frequent feeling of urination. All these symptoms could be indicative of a prostate problem.

THINK PREVENTION ABOUT
FEMALE-RELATED MATTERS

THE LOSS OF the uterus must be one of the most chilling possibilities a woman can face. The death of a person's libido and the warmth that accompanies it is a scary feeling when the woman is aware of its ultimate consequences. And yet, every day in America women are convinced to give away this priceless possession that the Creator gave them. The uterus and ovaries were given to the woman to perpetuate the human species. These were also given to her so that she could satisfy her natural need and the natural need of the opposite sex.

I know it isn't easy for a woman to experience unnecessary pain and extreme hemorrhaging as a result of fibrous tumors in the uterus or female reproductive tract. However, every naturopathic doctor or physician would want every woman and family member to know that having a hysterectomy should only be a last resort to avoid excruciating pain or death. Every day women are being treated for fibrous tumors with herbal supplements, proper diet, exercise, cleansing, and other stress-reducing methods with great success. Addressing the problem early with herbs and organ cleansing is of the utmost importance. Too often women procrastinate in the face of the problem, and it makes it more difficult to address later. Herbal remedies have been used for ages to correct female problems, which means there is hope outside of the removal of the female organs.

How is one to prevent such female problems from developing? We have found that improper diet and the lack of internal organ cleansing are the two main culprits. The proper working of the hormonal structure of the female endocrine system depends upon a program of balanced nutrition. Estrogen is an essential female hormone that naturally recedes as the female body ages. It helps to regulate the emotional temperament and biological constitution of the female. It helps keep the female motherly and womanly in conjugal matters. It helps make her feminine and warm. When the ovaries are damaged with cysts, tumors, or toxic waste, then the production of female hormones are affected. If you remove the ovaries, then the woman will lose some of the production of these hormones, thereby decreasing the libido.

Testimonials from women who have undergone this type of operation are distressing. Some say that this procedure can affect a woman's desire for a husband's touch, the feeling of sexual expression, the psychological uncertainty of the marriage relationship, mood swings, and emotional stability.

Surgery sometimes becomes necessary if one waits too long to address the symptoms or fails in prevention. After surgery, how is one to handle the outcome? The best thing is to accept that the surgery was the most helpful thing for that person. And although these people may not function the way they would like, they can still keep some balance in their lives. It is best to remain as nonjudgmental as possible. Don't question whether this development was good or bad, right or wrong. It just happened that way. It is not the end of the person's life, but the beginning of dealing with his or her life from another perspective. Husbands and other family members should also take the nonjudgmental approach.

When the diet contains too many bad elements such as sugar, caffeine, saturated fat, meat containing steroids and artificial hormones, white flour products, sodas, and other junk foods, the tissue structure in the female reproductive track becomes vulnerable to irritation. If not properly taken care of, this irritation will lead to inflammation, infection, ulceration, and possibly cancer.

The breast tissue is the same type of tissue that is present in the uterine tract. That's why it's susceptible to tumors. The constitutional strength of the tissue in the reproductive tract has to do with how fast the tissue will break down under the influence of toxic material and unhealthy elements. If there is a history of fibroids in the family, then a woman must be careful about her diet and cleansing habits. She could have an inherent weakness in the same tissue as her parents. However, this does not mean that one will automatically get fibroids, but it does mean one should be extremely careful about his or her habits.

At the time of menopause, the body has a tendency to go through changes. It is almost necessary to supplement the diet with nutrients that will balance the hormonal structure of the body. Night sweats, emotional stress, and hot flashes are some of the symptoms one may experience. Herbs such as black cohosh, red raspberry, and dong quai have been used with great success. However, you may want to contact a practitioner before using these. Using combinations of these herbs seems to give the best results. For prevention and care, I strongly recommend you use my body chemistry support system, three and seven day cleanse liver gallbladder flush to help bring about optimal results.

THE FEMALE AND THE HERB
RED RASPBERRY LEAF

T HE HERBAL KINGDOM is heavily laden with plants of all types with properties designed by Allah (God) to prevent pain and disease. We have known about many of these herbs and their abilities for ages, perhaps since the first man, Adam, and his wife. History tells us that Hippocrates, the father of Western medicine, was an herbalist. Botanical history tells us that during his time, only 235 herbs were known on the island of Cos in Asiatic Turkey, but with a selected few, he helped heal many people and others in the surrounding nations.

According to history, when Rome witnessed Hippocrates's success, she banished her allopathic physicians for six hundred years, and during that time the people recovered their health. Hippocrates, so it is written, didn't know anatomy and physiology, and he didn't know that the blood circulated through the body. And yet he is and has been held in the mind of Western medicine as the greatest physician to have ever lived. Incidentally, he was a student of Imhotep, an African.

In the category of astringent herbs, the wild red raspberry herb has to be one of nature's gifts to females because of its benefits to her urogenital system. Most everyone has eaten scrumptious pies and preserves made from its fruit, but most don't know that its leaves can make childbirth nearly painless.

Throughout history midwives have been known to give red raspberry tea with a little composition powder as the only drink during labor with great success in deliveries. Midwives have said that even if the child isn't coming out right during the birthing process, they can administer the tea, and the baby will turn and facilitate a speedy delivery. This is a herb that works on the female reproductive organs by toning, stimulating, and regulating them more efficiently than any other known herb. Red raspberry is a great gift for mothers and babies, and all women should know about it.

Red raspberry has been known to treat dysmenorrhea (painful menstruation) and amenorrhea (scanty menstruation). This herb has helped many women overcome pain and other discomfort during their monthly cycle with consistency. It is a wonderful herb to give to young girls at the time of puberty. Women don't have to experience trouble with menstruation if they take some red raspberry.

Both the leaves and the berries contain iron citrate. The production of blood as well as the astringent and contraction activity of the female organs and other internal tissues depend on iron citrate. The leaves also contain pectin, malic acid, and other organic acids, which carry oxygen to the cells. In addition, they carry calcium chloride, potassium chloride, and potassium sulfate. This is a great herb for women. The fruit contains iron, potassium, calcium salts of malic, and tartaric acid.

In his book *Advanced Treaties in Herbology*, Dr. Edward E. Shook states, "It has been used extensively and successfully in all female disorders, diarrhea, dysentery, cholera infantum, leucorrhea, Prolapsus uteri, Prolapsus ani, hemorrhoids, nausea of pregnancy, dyspepsia, vomiting of weak children." Red raspberry is known to prevent miscarriage, prevent afterbirth pains, enrich mother's milk, remove thrush, and treat urinary complaints, colds, and fevers. How could one herb do so many things? First, it's because Allah is gracious, and second, it's because of its chemical constituents.

The plant kingdom is abundant with medicinal herbs that are there to satisfy all our health needs. One herb can have various medicinal uses. For example, red raspberry is an astringent, tonic, homeostatic, antiseptic, antiabortient (prevents natural abortion), parturient, helps offset sexually transmitted disease, and its antimalarial. Every woman should use this herb to help her stay youthful, retain her health, and strengthen the genitalia.

The value of red raspberry cannot be overstated. I have always advocated that people find herbs that address their particular needs and consistently use them. Well, this is one of those herbs that every woman needs to use irrespective of age or condition.

RITALIN: OVERPRESCRIBED

Hyperactivity, lack of concentration and attention deficit disorder (ADD) are being diagnosed more often in schoolchildren today than ever before. In fact, since the advent of the drugs Dexedrine and Ritalin, it seems every schoolchild is prescribed Ritalin as the remedy for these conditions. The American school system is riddled with entire classes filled with children using Ritalin.

Conventionally, children who are hyperactive are treated with these drugs. Think about that. Your child might be on drugs for the first five or six years of his of her life, even though these drugs can have side effects that might do permanent harm. And no one knows the long-term side effects for children. Pharmaceutical companies will admit that Ritalin is a form of speed, but the children who are hyperactive are slowed down by it.

It's rare that these children are ever evaluated for nutritional, environmental, and food sensitivities, which all too often prove to be the cause in ADD. Because dietary restrictions are extremely difficult to handle for doctors, parents, and children, many don't take that route to control the problem. I lay the blame on those parents and doctors who know that food sensitivities could be the cause but opt to take the path of least resistance by putting their children or patients on drugs five days a week. Why wouldn't doctors investigate all possible causes before starting child patients on these controlled substances? And shouldn't parents do the same?

Foods such as sugar and bicarbonates are the main culprits in hyperactivity. Each morning parents give their children cereals and drinks that are loaded with sugar before they leave for school. On the way to school, children may even stop at the candy store or the corner bakery for gum, candy, sodas, doughnuts, and sweet rolls. Mix this sugar with a TV program like *The Three Stooges, Psycho, The Dark Side*, or some other programming depicting violence and fear, and you have a child who's hyperactive and won't let you rest. Then the child is prescribed Ritalin.

The average American eats up to 210 pounds of sugar per year. Because some of us don't eat as much as others, that means some people eat 250 to 300 pounds per year. That's alarming. That much sugar can produce an allergic reaction, and in most people it will cause adrenal gland burnout and diabetic conditions.

In a British publication called the *Lancet*, one author states,

> 185 hyperkinetic (Lack of concentration) children went on a low allergy diet of water, lamb and chicken, potatoes and rice, bananas and pears, cabbage, cauliflower, broccoli, cucumber, celery, and carrots. The diet was supplemented with calcium, magnesium, zinc, and vitamins. Behavior responded to food on both challenges, and elimination in 116 children. Forty of these children received intradermal hypersensitization, or placebo, and it was found that 16 of the 20 who received hypo sensitization could tolerate the foods after treatment. Hyperkinetic behavior was eliminated as long as the offending foods were avoided.

This study shows that all hyperkinetic children don't need to take Ritalin or any other drug. As a public, we need to make food allergy testing a requirement before any child is prescribed serious drugs.

As a parent, you must not underestimate the power of prayer and meditation to calm the mind and alleviate hyperactivity. Encourage your child to get up consistently in the morning for prayer before going to school. This will relieve some stress in the morning and give one a brighter outlook on the day's activities. Before you let doctors give your children Ritalin, examine their diet and think about other environmental factors that could lead to ADD and hyperactivity. Start there when you're looking for ways to correct the problem. You will be happy you did. Ritalin is overprescribed.

ASPIRIN: WHAT YOU THINK IT IS BUT MORE

S TATISTICS TELL US approximately twenty million pounds of aspirin are sold in the United States alone each year. More than fifteen tons of aspirin are consumed hourly. It has been manufactured to address pain of all types, including arthritis and headaches. It is used on such an ongoing basis because (1) aspirin is inexpensive, (2) it's easily available without prescription, (3) most believe that aspirin isn't habit forming, and (4) it makes one feel more comfortable by easing pain. Because of these reasons, aspirin is used each day on a massive scale, and it has become a habitual routine for suffers of arthritis, headaches, backaches, and other pains. Arthritic suffers and other users use it in increasing amounts, and many become so dependent on aspirin that they can hardly live without the drug. People need to be informed about how much damage this so-called *harmless* drug is doing to them on a daily basis.

Among health practitioners, there is a general agreement that aspirin is a toxic drug with many side effects. On November 15, 1947, the *Journal of the American Medical Association* stated that aspirin, which is technically known as acetylsalicylic acid, along with many other patented drugs that feature aspirin as the main ingredient, can cause severe poisoning and result in pathological changes in the brain, liver, and kidneys. The ingredients of the drug are still the same today. Used over a long period of time, aspirin is known to destroy agents of the immune system that promote the healing properties in the human body.

Aspirin has the ability to cover up symptoms in the acute stage of illness, and the problem gradually becomes more chronic through protracted use.

The *Journal of the American Medical Association* has also reported that even small doses of aspirin can cause cardiac weakness with an excessive pulse rate, edematous swelling of the mucus membrane, irregular pulse, and occasionally albuminuria (albumin in urine).

Aspirin is also reported to be antagonistic to many vitamins, especially vitamin C. It is reported that it destroys huge amounts of vitamin C while it's in the body. Its toxic side effects contribute to bleeding and blood thinning. Pregnant women and hemophiliacs have been warned against using it. It also has toxic side effects, including delirium and states of incoherence, restlessness, and confusion. Aspirin is not the harmless drug many have portrayed it to be.

Aspirin is an analgesic, which only means it can relieve pain. There are natural herbs that are pain-relieving or analgesic in nature that don't carry such side effects, such as black and white willow. These herbs are used daily throughout the world by wise people who suffer with pain. Black and white willow are natural aspirins that are nontoxic. They are used to address inflammation and pain. They reduce fever, and they target the nervous system. They are good for internal and external use. The bark of the plant is used as well, and it may be referred to as willow bark or as salix nigra and salix alba in homeopathic remedies.

Herbal alignment, which consists of the combination of capsicum and Indian tobacco, is a marvelous remedy for back and joint pain, headaches, heart problems, and circulation issues. You can apply this externally on the back and joints with peppermint oil. It targets the circulatory system.

Clove, known as a (caryophyllus aromatic), is used in homeopathic remedies, and it is a great pain reliever. It's often used for pain relief, especially toothaches. It is good for nausea and cramping, and it destroys the eggs of parasites and cysts. It targets all the body systems also. The unopened flower buds are dried and then used. These are some natural remedies, and there are even more that deal with pain that could easily replace aspirin at any time.

In many cases, we would do ourselves a great service if we looked for alternatives to many of the traditional drugs that have aspirin in them today. However, if you have persistent pains, contact a health practitioner. If you still have the pain after that, try someone else. Don't give up. There could be permanent relief for your pain. When you become wiser and stronger about your own health, you can make life more comfortable for yourself.

POOR NUTRITION AND MARITAL AFFAIRS

T ODAY, TOO MANY people are headed for religious leaders or some other counselor's office for marital advice. The threat of divorce and the dissolution of relationships may be a more prevalent thing today than ever before. It seems that with so much knowledge available and the testimonies of other people's experiences—good or bad—we should have a better understanding of marital relationships and what will preserve and sustain them. And while mass media and bad examples are usually the culprits in these failed relationships, I submit that poor diet is also a contributing factor.

Most people usually don't perform well when they don't feel well. When the nerves are not fed with the proper nutrients, people seem to always be on edge, and this can lead to explosive tempers, snap judgments, or unnecessary social friction. When a person is in this mode, the entire family is at risk of being scolded. When a person can't move their bowels and constipation has set in, he or she doesn't feel well, and this affects his or her attitude in a negative way. Indigestion, extreme fatigue syndrome, insomnia, and other ailments are all factors influencing how we relate to others. When humans are in pain, it doesn't matter how favorable their social circumstances may be. They don't enjoy the atmosphere at all, and if they are not careful, they won't let others enjoy those good circumstances either. While I know there can be other factors in the destruction of vital relationships, I believe it's first how we feel personally and second how we feel about the matter that leads to the dissolution of the relationship or the social friction.

As humans, we must become more conscious of our diets and how they affect our performance if we are to maintain our vital relationships.

An article published by *Fit Today* (November 19, 2017) states, "Caffeine has been known to disrupt the proper function of a person's nerves." Too much sugar will make us hypersensitive. Too much bread and meat will make us constipated. These are some of the factors that can lead to a bad attitude. The cook in the home must be mindful that what he or she puts on the table at mealtime can and will regulate the environmental factors in the home. Most humans usually eat what is put before them at mealtime. If obesity is a common concern in your family, why perpetuate a diet that makes you prone to gaining weight. If the diet isn't in your or your family's best interest, you must help change the diet for the sake of your health and the health of those you love. *Learn to cook for health and taste, and gradually supplement and change the diet.* It will take your will, courage, and determination to improve their health, but you can if you want to.

Imam W. Deen Mohammed pointed out at an imams' meeting in Harvey, Illinois, that we should be careful of foods that are converted into sugar inside the body, such as potatoes and navy beans, because they can lead to diabetic conditions. The imam suggested we look at the fermented soybean, which is higher in protein and would not contribute to this deadly disorder. Imam W. Deen Mohammed is correct. We must begin to look at other foods that many of us are not accustomed to, scrutinize them, and incorporate them into our diets for health purposes. Experience has shown that these foods, including fermented soy products, can be prepared so that they taste as good as or better than the foods that are leading to the problems.

Don't give up and say, "I can't change. And the family doesn't want the change," when you know that your present diet isn't contributing to better health. That will only lead to poor health and bigger marital and family problems. Ask people you know who are health-conscious what a good book for you to read would be if you think asking them to help you learn to cook in a new way will be too much of an imposition for them.

It would be good to start nutrition and healthy cooking classes in our houses of worship along with all the other classes. The community's health is of the utmost importance. Dear religious leader, you must take the lead in building better health in the religious community. Good health has become one of your personal priorities, and you should make it a collective priority for your immediate public. This is a must if you want this generation to improve in their health and the next generation to come up healthy. We should not lose the battle on the field of health.

I believe we can cut down on some of the marital problems if we can improve how people feel. Sometimes a husband will say to a wife or vice versa, "The reason you are acting like this is because you don't believe the Good Book." This is not always true. In some cases, because of health issues, a person is just not up to what you are proposing. I think we should always question whether a person's heart and mind can handle what we are. Before we make a decision that is going to affect a person, make sure you talk it over. Sometimes the nerves are just too weak to handle various matters, and at times like that, it has nothing to do with belief.

When my wife, Connie, and I were considering having our last child, she said, "I have to consider my health first," and she was right. Well, my daughter, Intisar, was a healthy arrival, and Connie was fine during the pregnancy and after delivery. However, in the decision-making process, her health was our first priority.

"What can I do about my husband's snoring or my snoring?" one may ask. "He thinks I don't want to sleep with him when the real reason I sleep on the couch is we both snore very loud and I can't sleep." First, let him know you still love him, then ask him to seek professional help for his respiratory problem. His poor eating habits, lack of exercise, and lack of cleansing over the years has probably led to this problem. Say to him, "I want to be able to sleep with you more often, so let's work on the problem." Ask him if he would be willing to change his diet if it would help. If he says yes, seek counseling on a new diet that will lend itself to respiratory health and a lack of snoring. The wife should follow the same process.

"Is there anything my spouse and I can use to improve our sexual relationship?" one may ask. As religious people, we should first understand that Allah (God) has ordained the purpose of marital sex as procreation. In addition, it is difficult for people to believe that they are not supposed to enjoy their partners in a sexual way. The release of stress and tension that we derive from the sexual act has the human being desiring its expression and fulfillment naturally. Sex is healthy for us physically and morally. It is not a sin, and it is healthy for our soul. When a couple isn't enjoying each other in this manner, one of the easiest things to question first is diet. In the female, the body's ability to regulate its hormones determines readiness or frigidity. In most cases, when a woman is feeling cold about sex, it is a biological matter that can be resolved with nutrients and minor lifestyle changes. That lack of passion may be in your mind, but it could also be coming from an imbalance in your body.

In regards to sex, a woman wants a man to express the feminine side of his soul too. Contrary to what most men have been taught, if the male cannot stimulate the feminine side of his soul while he's engaged in sex, he will not give his wife her greatest fulfillment. Putting food on the table is masculine; satisfying your wife sexually is feminine. Women want romance in their lives, and if the hormones in the male aren't balanced, he is not warm in romantic or sexual matters. Sisters, you may see this coldness through his mental expression, but it could be a nutritional deficiency first. Nutritional deficiencies will lead to these problems that can affect otherwise healthy marital relations. There are nutrients that both males and females can use to improve sexual relations. Don't be ashamed to recommend to your spouse something you think will enhance your sexual relations. Allah will reward you for it. Nutrition plays a major part in the equation of happiness in our marriages, so don't overlook it.

SOMETIMES YOUR BODY NEEDS A COLD

DESPITE WHAT WE may think when we get a cold, it may be what our body needs to cleanse itself of unwanted toxic material. During the fall and winter seasons, it is commonplace for many people to get colds or contract the flu virus because the conditions are ripe for these illnesses in their bodies. However, the germ theory is still being perpetrated in the public, suggesting that a germ is all that is required to develop these illnesses. ABC News recently announced that there were various cities in these United States that were vulnerable to a flu virus, so the people in those cities should brace themselves for the invasion. The reality is that if people in any of these cities do not have the right conditions present in their bodies, they will not get a cold or the flu. No one would get a cold if the immune response was high enough to ward off infection and the body was clean and free of the virus. I'm not saying that a virus has nothing to do with a cold. What I am saying is that the virus that could cause a cold is harmless to you if the defense system is nutrient-based. People primarily fall ill because they are nutrient-deficient and/or they are filled with excessive toxins.

What is the flu, and where does it come from? The flu is a buildup of toxic material that presents as a cold as the body tries to eliminate it, but the person usually doesn't let the mucus flow reach its completion. When you get a cold, you often go to the doctor or druggist and get an antibiotic to suppress the flow or relieve yourself of the unwanted feeling. Then that undigested protein that the body is trying to rid itself of remains in the body. Plus, the antibiotic consumed will accumulate in the body. If you reach for antibiotics each time you get a cold, then in time you will get the flu. If this pattern continues, it will ultimately build disease in the body.

Building disease in your body is a process. It starts with a common cold. Suppressing a cold continuously will lead to the flu. Suppressing the flu with antibiotics will lead to a cough. Suppressing a cough with a cough suppressant (antibiotic) will lead to bronchitis, which is an inflamed condition of the lungs. Using antibiotics or other immune-suppressant drugs for bronchitis will lead to pneumonia. Using antibiotics for pneumonia will lead to emphysema or some other inherent health problem. Using antibiotics for emphysema will lead to cancer. With this pattern, cancer may be found or detected at the end of the process anywhere in the body. This is so because the toxic material always gravitates to where there is an inherent weakness in the body.

People often inherit weaknesses in tissues from their parents. If the liver was weak, cancer may be found in the liver at the end of the process. It's the same with the spleen, kidneys, stomach, lungs, etc. There is no cure for a cold. The cold is the cure. And the process starts when one suppresses the cold.

Research shows that taking herbs, vitamin C, rose hips, or any other immune system stimulant that is designed to build the immune response at the first signs of a cold is better than taking antibiotics. However, if the lack of cellular cleansing that brought the cold isn't changed, it will surface again in the future. If you don't voluntarily submit to a cleanse, then the body will subject you to an involuntary one in time.

Your Creator has given the body the ability to endure the common cold, which is really a necessary purging process. However, good eating habits, regular cleansing, rest, exercise, and wholesome thinking is what the Creator prescribed for man. We should seek prevention before cure. However, you should always remember that sometimes your body needs a cold.

GOOD HEALTH DEPENDS UPON
PROPER DIGESTION

M OST PEOPLE DON'T know their bodies weren't designed to digest all their foods. The foods we consume should themselves assist in their own digestion so that our bodies don't have to do all the work. All raw foods have predigestive enzymes in them. Nature put the enzymes to digest or decompose the food in each item in order to keep the ecological order in balance. If things did not decompose when they died, we would have dead carcasses all over the planet. However, the enzymes that are necessary to digest the food are destroyed during the cooking process. Therefore, most people are using all their internal enzymes to digest their foods, which takes away energy from other important functions of the body, such as healing, excretion, secretion, and elimination. We should eliminate the extreme depletion of our internal enzymes by using digestive enzymes with each meal. Enzymes are often referred to as the spark of life. There can be no life without enzymatic activity.

Every living thing has enzymes to support its life. The human body is born with an enzyme bank for metabolic and digestive purposes. Humans are born with a limited amount of amylase to digest starch and a limited amount of protease to digest protein.

And we need lipase to digest fats. Every time our body uses some of these inborn enzymes, we deplete the bank. Humans can eat so much cooked food or live enzyme-deficient food that in time our bodies won't have sufficient energy to digest our food. Then we won't be able to enjoy life without popping a pill to get rid of indigestion. Without enzymes, gases develop, and acids are left unchecked in the alimentary canal. This all leads to discomfort and inconvenience.

There are thousands of processes in the body that are affected by different enzymes. Metabolic enzymes are different from food enzymes in the way they act in and on the body. Nevertheless, they are all important in the body's life processes.

Humans replenish their bodies by eating enzyme-rich foods or foods that still have live enzymes in them. Ptyalin or saliva enzymes have the ability to release the enzymes from the food after ingestion and mastication. My protein power, the Essential Light, nutritious drink, and plant enzymes are loaded with enzymes in their raw state. I highly recommend my meal pack for organic minerals and vitamins each day. In most cases, raw foods will be better for our bodies because they still have their life in them. However, because we eat so much cooked food, we should make a good habit of taking digestive enzymes at each meal to assist in the digestion of that meal. If we use digestive enzymes, we won't have to use our internal enzymes to break down our food, and in some cases, we may even be deficient of the necessary enzymes to break down the meal. Using digestive enzymes will retard the aging process and give us greater energy for other bodily processes.

DIABETES AND THE THINGS TO DO AND CONSIDER

JUVENILE OR TYPE 1 diabetes, normally found in children or youth, is seen as a true insulin-dependent form of diabetes, and it requires insulin to regulate blood sugar levels. This form of diabetes can be inherited, but in most cases, it comes from a diseased or toxic pancreas.

In type 2 diabetes, referred to as adult-onset diabetes, which is becoming more common in our youth because of modern lifestyles, the pancreas can produce sufficient insulin, but the cells don't respond to it. In normal cases, insulin will enter into the cells at receptor sites. However, when fat, cholesterol, and sugar plug these sites, they become insensitive to insulin, causing the sugar to remain in the bloodstream, which in turn causes hyperglycemia or high blood sugar. Insulin resistance is closely related to insulin insensitivity in that the body is producing enough insulin, but allergic reactions to certain foods keep insulin from doing its job.

Statistics say diabetes mellitus claims the lives of approximately 250,000 people per year in the United States alone. Medical reports also say that an increase in diabetes corresponds to an increase in heart disease. The underlying cause of the problem is the increase in the consumption of refined carbohydrates and saturated fats. That's why the onset of type 2 diabetes is more common than the juvenile type. It seems to be stimulated by a poor diet, a lack of exercise, and obesity. Basically, the beginning stages of type 2 diabetes are not noticeable since it doesn't present clear symptoms. Abdominal obesity is an indicator that possible diabetes is prevalent.

Today the method of treatment by allopathic physicians is more insulin, which has shown itself to be ineffective in 90 percent of the cases. In the juvenile form, additional insulin is needed because the body doesn't produce enough. But when the body is insensitive or resistant to insulin, the prescription of more insulin leads to kidney, heart failure, and even blindness. Hardening of the arteries has been directly related to the body's inability to handle excessive amounts of insulin.

Since the 1920s, when man-made insulin was first introduced, many children have extended their lives with its usage. Before that, insulin-dependent diabetic patients were given a poor outlook on the future, and blindness, gout, and gangrene were actually uncontrollable in juvenile diabetes.

The big concern with insulin is that it is prescribed in a universal context, not only to those who are insulin-deficient. When this hormone is given to a person who already has sufficient insulin, it does nothing to address the problem. In fact, its use becomes counterproductive. Insulin can stimulate a counteragent in the body that impedes its ability to lower blood sugar levels. When the blood sugar begins to fall as a result of the consumption of insulin, the body responds with an output of growth hormone and epinephrine. These hormones keep blood sugar levels elevated. Here, a rebound effect is the outcome of aggressive insulin therapy. Today we know that a constant fluctuation of blood sugar leads to all types of complications. Clinical studies show a 40 percent greater chance of eye problems in people with diabetes who are treated with aggressive insulin therapy than those treated moderately. Inner arterial wall damage and cardiovascular problems are also results of insulin treatment. Seventy-five percent of all deaths of diabetics are due to heart disease brought on by the hardening of major arteries.

CONGESTIVE HEART FAILURE

H EART FAILURE OCCURS when the heart can't pump enough blood to satisfy the needs of the other vital organs in the body. This condition can develop from coronary artery disease or narrowed arteries that supply blood to the heart muscle. High blood pressure, previous heart attack, or myocardial infarction can produce heart failure as well. Heart valve disease can come from past bouts of rheumatic fever, which can also affect the kidneys, and it can also be a contributing factor. Congenital heart disease or a defect in the heart that was present at birth is related to congestive heart failure as well. So too, heart failure can come as a result of an infection of the heart valves and muscle (or both).

When blood that flows out of the heart slows, the returning blood to the heart by way of the veins backs up, producing congestion in the tissue. Oftentimes edema (swelling) occurs in the ankles and the legs. However, it could happen in other parts of the body. Sometimes fluid will develop in the lower respiratory tract or lungs and interfere with breathing, particularly when a person is lying down, causing shortness of breath. This leads to the heart working below normal, and it also doesn't work as efficiently as it should. It is challenging for people with these conditions to exert themselves because of this shortness of breath and fatigue.

Heart failure also affects the kidneys in that they lose their ability to dispose of sodium and water, and this excess water increases the swelling.

The most common symptoms of congestive heart failure are swollen legs or ankles as well as difficulty breathing. Weight gain because of the buildup of fluid is also usually present.

Congestive heart failure requires a treatment program of rest, proper diet, modified activities, cellular cleansing, good nutrition, and enzyme therapy. Herbs such as corn silk, uva ursi, and gravel root all address fluid retention and support the kidneys.

Motherwort, hawthorn, myrrh, and capsicum strengthen the heart muscle, valves, and blood vessels. They also lower blood pressure, address palpitations, and regulate heartbeat. Coltsfoot, elecampane, blessed thistle, comfrey, bugleweed, and yerba santa remove fluid from around the heart and lungs. Coenzyme Q10 is an antioxidant in nature and strengthens the heart. These and many more herbs that are comprised of organic minerals, essential fatty acids, essential amino acids, cellulose, and antioxidants will address congestive heart failure. For information about the proper amounts for your body, please call my office or see your health practitioner.

When you discover the causes of your congestive heart failure, you should address it and correct your lifestyle immediately if possible. Oftentimes treating high blood pressure will correct heart failure. The most drastic approach is surgery. If one waits too long to address the symptoms, then the heart can't be repaired by the body's self-healing mechanisms. Most cases of mild to moderate heart failure can be treated with proper supervision. Please don't wait to contact a health practitioner if you are experiencing some of the symptoms.

A CLEAN BLOOD CULTURE IS INSURANCE

T HE HUMAN BODY must have a clean blood culture for good health. This comes first in the body's ability to digest food and eliminate waste. The body has a natural respiration (energy making system) to it that ensures its health. Consuming clean air, water, and food is vital in this process. In addition, the elimination of unused food or waste after metabolism is also a part of the body's respiratory process. When elimination is not in proportion to consumption, then the body's overall respiration process will be disturbed, and cellular fatigue will follow.

A high fiber diet will give the body a chance to breathe properly by expediting elimination. Regular exercise is indispensable, and it will also add to the body's consumption of oxygen and give our body more effective respiration.

The colon is the body's sewage system. As in any sewage system, if it's not kept open and clean, then complications will arise. For example, if we permit the toilets in our houses to become congested with waste that should ultimately end up outside the house in the city's sewage system, then the health of those in the house will be put in jeopardy. A lack of elimination because of constipation or compacted, unexpelled waste also puts the person at risk because the waste cannot be reabsorbed by a healthy bloodstream. The body must be clean to ensure health. The bloodstream carries the nutrients and waste to and from the cells. The blood represents the prevalent culture of the body. Its cleanliness (or lack thereof) is critical to the overall health of the entire organism. The first step to having a clean culture or bloodstream in the body is having a clean bowel.

If everything that went into the body was eliminated expeditiously after digestion or if bowel movements occur within twelve to twenty-four hours, there would be no serious need for conscious voluntary cleansing or colonics and enemas. However, this is not always the case. Undigested foods have a tendency to become trapped in the body when the colon muscle is restricted. Low fiber intake, inadequate amounts of water, a lack of exercise and rest, and lower back muscle congestion are all primary reasons for the entrapment of most foods. As a result, the unexpelled food spoils, rots, and becomes toxic. The bloodstream carries it to all the cells in the body, and it leads to serious fatigue among other things. The cells in the body must function properly to make energy and generate heat so that the entire body can have optimal health.

The act of conversion (digestion) or the lack of conversion of raw material (nutrient-rich food) into a usable form is responsible for the growth, maturity, and death of the organism.

Metabolism primarily involves two aspects—anabolism and catabolism. Anabolism has to do with the process of building up, and catabolism has to do with the processes of disintegration or tearing down. Anabolism is the process of converting ingested elements into parts of protoplasm or the basis of all living activities (e.g., assimilation, growth, secretion, and reproduction). Catabolism is the process of breaking down substances into fundamental parts, and the results are then excreted in most cases. These processes work better in a clean culture or environment when the blood is healthy. Order my body chemistry support system today, and start the process of detoxifying the blood and ensuring good health.

THERE IS NO OPTION TO GOOD HEALTH

THE YOUNGER HUMAN beings are, the more they take good health for granted. And yet the older we get, the more we realize that enjoying this life in its fullness depends heavily on optimal health. The need or want of good health is not an option to be considered by humans when we are faced with the reality of human life. The infinite intelligence has placed in our souls a natural inclination for health even if we see all other people in our environment sick. In our best state of mind, we don't want to be sick, even if our loved ones are. Our nervous system naturally moves us away from pain toward pleasure.

Yesterday's habits have produced today's health, and today's habits will produce tomorrow's health. The only way we can overcome the fear of sickness in the future is by developing new habits that produce health today. Health and sickness are based on the natural law of cause and effect. Good habits of regular exercise and rest will help tremendously in preserving our health. If our diets consist of plenty of clean water and nutrients, our bodies will be healthy. Poor habits of exercise and rest, not consuming enough clean water, and neglecting proper nutrition will produce a weak body that is susceptible to sickness.

If you want to have good health, exercise is a must. Rest and relaxation are incredibly important, and maintaining proper nutrition is a must. These are not options.

What is more important—your schedule or your health? What is more important—money or your health? Is it more important that you live a healthy life with your family or that they are forced to live without you? Don't let your ignorance contribute to your destruction. Educate yourself and take action.

I love pancakes with blueberries and honey, turkey sausage, eggs, and oatmeal. I could eat that breakfast perhaps three times per week. However, I realize that this meal consists of a lot of calories, which means I must burn them in exercise. If I don't, the food will produce fat. So too, there aren't a lot of good nutrients or predigestive enzymes in this meal, so I must supplement them with this meal. This will help preserve my health. Approximately thirty minutes after the meal, I need at least one eight-ounce glass of clean water to assist in digestion and to prevent dehydration of the internal organs. If you practice the principles of good health, you can eat almost anything you choose that your body can digest. However, if you overeat and fail to implement these health principles, you run the risk of sickness.

It is foolish to think that you can eat red meats, poultry, fish, potatoes, pasta, breads, sweets, and cooked foods and have good health without burning these calories with strenuous exercise. Hypertension, diabetes, cancer, and obesity are all related to a lack of exercise and exertion. The body has been built to endure heavy exertion when it is healthy. It can endure more exercise than what most people think. Start today, and exercise your body regularly until you can experience the pleasure of exhaustion after your workout. When you reach that point, you are well on your way to good health. Doesn't it stand to reason that athletes get pleasure out of exercise? Why would they do it otherwise?

The stronger you make your body, the better it will handle stress. The stronger you make your body, the faster the recovery time and more work it can endure. The weaker the body is, the more rest you need, the longer the recovery time after excursion, and the more susceptible you are to stress.

Good nutrition, exercise, and rest are the keys to optimal health. There are no options for good health in this life.

THE DEVELOPMENT OF DISEASE AND
BEING MINDFUL OF ANTIBIOTICS

L ET ME SHOW you how the suppression of the so-called common cold through the use of antibiotics leads to many of the serious disorders we face today, such as cardiovascular problems, cancer, diabetes, obesity, and arthritis, among others.

When the human body can't tolerate any additional undigested foods and unused foodstuff, the body's systems begin an elimination process of the mucus or catarrh that develops from poor digestion, which expresses itself as what we call the common cold. Modern medicine has discovered how to manufacture a medicine called antibiotics that will stop the flow of this mucus. In America, we are better at creating disease than most nations on the earth today. Antibiotics may appear to help the patient, but in a way that isn't obvious, they are contributing to disease in the long run. The seemingly immediate relief from the common cold, flu, aches, and pains carry the false message of health. In this case, the person begins to feel better, which falsely suggests that he or she is healthier now that the symptoms are gone. However, unknowing to the patient, the friendly bacteria in the gastrointestinal tract has been destroyed. As a result, various harmful bacteria and viruses that were once held in check by the good bacteria, which support the immune system, are unleashed. The friendly bacteria must be in the body in adequate amounts to ensure good health.

One must understand that it is automatic for the body to begin a natural, involuntary cleansing process if the person won't cleanse him- or herself voluntarily. However, humans don't want to feel uncomfortable or be inconvenienced, so when the involuntary cleanse begins, they reach for an antibiotic. If one persists with this behavior, in time it's the flu that becomes common for the person. This happens because the mucus that the body wanted to expel through the cold was forced to remain in the body. Additionally, the influx of the antibiotics builds to the point of infection and the irritation of the tissue as the immune response is lowered.

If one continues to follow the same habits of overeating, lack of rest, lack of cleansing, and other bad habits that lead to the immune response becoming weaker, the person will ultimately develop a cough, sinus infection, or other possible respiratory problems. These problems will nag the person until he or she feels it necessary to go to the doctor, again seeking another antibiotic or a cough suppressant. Through this cough the body is trying to expel the unwanted, undigested mucus plus the previous antibiotic.

As the body degenerates under the suppression of natural cleansing, it will degenerate next to bronchitis, pneumonia, emphysema, and ultimately cancer. People must ask themselves, "How can I stop this process?" Here are ways you can cease this process:

1. Replenish the body with friendly bacteria, such as lactobacillus acidophilus and bifidus.
2. Make sure that you cleanse the large bowel every few months and use herbal supplements to rid the body of parasites.
3. Increase the consumption of dietary fiber by supplementing up to twenty-five to fifty grams daily.
4. Drink at least six to eight eight-ounce glasses of clean water each day, preferably slightly alkaline water.
5. Make sure you get adequate rest.
6. Exercise at least three times per week for approximately twenty minutes.
7. Be careful of antibiotic use and restrict their use totally if possible.

If you believe in the Creator, you should trust His natural creation to support your health. Nature has the largest pharmacy. You simply need education, and you must use your intuition today. Our parents trusted and used nature's plants when there weren't any man-made drugs. We should study the plant and mineral kingdoms and use their healing agents.

A SPECIAL KEY: CLEANSING THE COLON

THE NOTION THAT cleansing the colon will somehow relieve disorders or rejuvenate the human organism is not new. As far back as human beings can remember, purgatives to relieve stomachaches and constipation, such as hydrated bentonite, aloe vera, cascara sagrada, senna leaf, and castor oil, have been used as remedies to expel unwanted waste. This waste of undigested matter, mostly composed of proteins, leads to the development of catarrh, which in turn leads to discharge, the common cold, or the beginning of disease.

For many years of my youth and adult life, I suffered with constipation. I didn't have the slightest idea why my body was tired and sluggish so often. It wasn't until I met a naturopathic doctor who was also a practicing iridologist that I found out about all the old fecal matter that was trapped in my body. After subjecting myself to a series of colonics, high enemas, and colon cleansing herbs, I felt so much better. My energy level improved and unhealthy sinus symptoms faded away. The reality is that most people today are walking around with pounds of this putrid matter in their bowels. Some studies say a person could have more than thirty to fifty pounds of this unwanted putrid matter in his or her body.

The need to remove this morbid matter from the body is so crucial to improved health that most alternative health care practitioners recommend it as one of the first steps in rejuvenating lost health. It is also suggested as a consistent measure to maintain a healthy balance between body, mind, and spirit.

THE PRIMITIVE GUT TUBE

ONE OF THE first things to develop in the embryo in the womb of its mother is the primitive gut tube. We can see this tube with budding developments after approximately four weeks of growth. Ultimately, this tube becomes the large bowel, large intestine, and/or colon, and these shapes that look like buds become organs that make up the human body. As the gut tube grows into the colon, these organs remain attached to the colon via the nervous system.

Through this development, we can see the importance of cleansing the colon. If our vital organs have a direct relationship with the colon through the nervous system, it is imperative to maintain the health of the colon to protect these vital organs. The flow from the colon to these organs and glands, as well as the flow from the organs and glands to the colon, is critical to the effective functioning of the organs and systems in the body. When the colon becomes congested with fecal matter, then nerve stimulation to and from these vital organs is lost, leading to imbalance and improper cellular function. Many operations on the colon for one purpose have accidentally cleared up other problems. The doctors have reported that operating on a patient for diverticulitis or colon cancer many times has led to the cleaning of parts of the colon that were not directly affected, and in doing so kidney and liver problems went away after the operation.

This tells us that restricted nerve flow from a congested colon will affect the efficient functioning of organs and glands in other parts of the body. Therefore, we should pay attention to the colon since its cleansing is clearly linked to the prevention of disease in the body. This attention will also lead to the activation of the body's own healing powers. If most people knew that their heart, stomach, adrenal glands, eyes, prostate, ovaries, and other vital organs and glands were all linked in the gut, they would take better care of it. The body can heal itself if it is given a chance through proper maintenance. One of the main factors in this maintenance is cleansing the colon.

SPRING: THE TIME TO CLEANSE
AND DETOX THE LIVER

A T THE COMMENCEMENT of each spring, cleansing the liver is one of the most prudent things human beings can do. I look forward to the day when a large numbers of Americans will engage in internal organ cleansing at prescribed times of the year without notice. It will be a great time for health in our nation, and I believe it will start to happen for many in the near future.

The liver is the largest organ in the human body. It secretes bile, and it contains many metabolic functions. Situated next to the liver is the gallbladder, which is connected to the cystic and hepatic ducts or vessels. These form the common bile duct. This bile duct enters the duodenum, which forms a part of your small intestine that's connected to your stomach. When the bile leaves the liver, it enters the gallbladder. There it is stored until the small intestine needs it for digestive purposes. The liver is also responsible for removing cellular debris, bacteria, and other foreign substances from the bloodstream. The liver's blood supply comes from the hepatic artery and portal vein. Think about what happens when these blood vessels are clogged with undigested fats and other substances. It short-circuits the entire network and leads to indigestion, gas, and poor elimination. The cellular body is ultimately starved of nutrients, and that leads to various diseases.

The liver is the first organ to receive a blood supply from the intestine. Eighty percent of the body's digestion takes place in the lower part of the small intestine. If the bile is not secreted by the gallbladder to start the process of digesting fats in the duodenum (upper part of the intestine), then the blood leaving the intestine will not have the nutrients to feed the cells.

Moreover, your nerve flow, energy levels, the manufacturing of proteins, and some hormonal functions depend upon a clean liver. The liver is the storage place for vitamin B12, which prevents anemia. It also stores the fat-soluble vitamins A, D, E, and K, which are antioxidants that help prevent damage from free radicals. These are all important in fat metabolism. The liver manufactures good cholesterol, which is found in most body cells and is also a major constituent of bile.

The liver is known as the organ of life and action. Spring is a time of new life. Relieve some of your body's stress by cleaning your liver and gallbladder. For more instructions, order my workbook by calling the office at 336-852-3040. Cleanse the liver, and enjoy the spring.

SUMMER: THE TIME TO CLEANSE AND DETOX
THE HEART AND ARTERIAL SYSTEM

D URING MY SEMINARS or my live television program, I am often asked what one can take for a particular ailment. People seem to think there is a single pill or quick fix that will act as a cure-all. Nothing from outside your body can heal your body. Anything from outside can only influence the body. In most cases, fitting illness takes a combination of influences, such as nutrition, good digestion, and good elimination. Then the body can heal itself. It is the intuitive wisdom of the body that is built into our cellular structure by our Creator that causes the body to heal itself. It is a self-healing mechanism that needs encouragement through the use of nutrients. Water, minerals, proteins, and nucleic acids all supports this mechanism for healing. Coupled with exercise, rest, and focused attention, this self-healing mechanism can help your body maintain quality health throughout your lifetime. Allah has been so merciful in His creation of our bodies (temples). On an instinctive level, they can recognize the raw materials that lead to the self-healing of your body. Ignorance of this self-healing mechanism can lead to complications in your body that will ultimately affect your health throughout your entire life. It is a natural law that prevails regardless of our personal likes and dislikes. It's not personal. It's universal.

I have found that physical and mental illness heavily influences toxicity levels. I must reiterate the importance of annual *intentional tissue cleansing*. Some people have called my office to ask about the arteries and heart cleansing at the start of each summer, and I have suggested my body chemistry support system in addition to an herbal formula. This is because most people are constipated or have been most of their lives. You may not be moving your bowels at least three times per day. If you are not constipated and your bowel is moving with regularity three times per day, then we can recommend herbal formulas without considering the entire body chemistry support system. However, with this summer cleanse recommendation, we hope you have done some intentional tissue cleansing in the past. If the bowel isn't moving with regularity, we advise the use of the body chemistry support system before you attempt the arteries and heart cleanse.

You should always consider how the bowel is moving before any cleanse. It won't be helpful if you release the waste material from a system or organ into the bloodstream or lymph system and it not be removed from the body. Remember—the liver and the gallbladder do not eliminate their waste directly from the body. The kidneys, skin, bowel, and the lungs do. However, when the waste is released from the tissue of any organ such as the heart muscle or the arterial walls, it will accumulate in the blood or lymph if not removed expeditiously. So the timely elimination of this accumulation of waste is necessary. Failing to act now may determine whenever you need surgery later or even die. Respect the Creator's laws and experience His mercy.

We should always think about processes when addressing our health from a natural standpoint. Remember there are no magic pills when it is time to detoxify and cleanse the arterial system and the heart.

FALL: THE TIME TO CLEANSE AND DETOX THE RESPIRATORY TRACK

A S WE ENTER the fall and colder conditions, we need to detoxify the respiratory tract of mucus and undigested protein to keep colds and flu away. Because most of us have been improperly combining our foods and eating processed, cooked, and lifeless food, the self-healing mechanisms of our bodies have been excreting mucus and storing it as toxic waste in the bowel to prevent it from circulating throughout the entire body. This is a natural process. The problem arises when we are at an extreme, and most people are. When the body can no longer tolerate the buildup of mucus from its own natural protecting processes, it creates a flow of the mucus or a cold. In time it will lead to the flu or an infection and ultimately cancer.

The respiratory tract, consisting of the bronchioles, lungs, throat, sinuses, and other parts, is the main track of elimination for the body. Mucus is consistently eliminated from the respiratory tract. You might often notice that after consuming processed, cooked, or improperly combined foods, you try to cough the mucus from the throat or blow it from the nostrils. This is telling you that you have a mild allergy to that food. The change in temperature acts as a trigger for the release of mucus. And sometimes during fasting the body will throw off the waste of undigested foodstuff. The fast will act as a trigger for the release of mucus. If a virus from another person gets the opportunity to express itself in your body it is because you have cultivated an environment in your body for its expression. Clean up the culture voluntarily, and viruses from other people lose their power to do you harm.

For respiratory cleansing I recommend you first cleanse the bowel and the lymphatic system and then use herbs that act as purgatives to remove mucus from the lungs, bronchioles, sinuses, and other organs. For a recommended program, call my office and ask for my respiratory cleansing pack.

WINTER: THE TIME TO DETOX AND CLEANSE THE KIDNEY

F OR SOME YEARS I have been talking about the importance of internal organ cleansing. At the commencement of the winter season, we highly recommend that people cleanse their kidneys to prevent kidney failure. More often than not these days, we hear about renal failure, dialysis, bladder infection, and other issues. Most of these disorders if not all of them are the result of innocent ignorance or willful neglect, and they are normally diet-related. Becoming more conscious of our diets and the proper working of our glands and organs in our bodies would be very helpful in preventing kidney dysfunction.

The kidneys excrete urine to help regulate the water, electrolyte, and acid-base content of the blood. Urine consists of water (95 percent) and solids (5 percent), and the latter should be in solution. The solids include urea, hippuric acid, uric acid, creatinine, and inorganic constituents, mainly salts of sodium and potassium. The kidneys remove these substances from the blood in an effort to maintain the balance of the blood and bodily fluids. Urine is formed through the process of filtration and reabsorption. When the kidneys are in their best condition, they can perform these functions optimally.

With chronic kidney disease, one can be at home treating themselves for kidney failure or going to the clinic for the use of the "Artificial," a machine or device that produces dialysis for the patient. This device uses dialysis to remove wastes from the blood just as the kidneys do. And after the process of filtration, it returns the blood to the patient. This artificial device used in treating patients with renal failure or absent kidney function does nothing to restore kidney function. Some patients must go to clinics at least three times per week for approximately three hours per visit to use this artificial device. A person's normal lifestyle becomes severely restricted. We know that inherited weaknesses can cause kidney complications; however, we believe annual cleansing can help offset tissue degeneration. Clients have come to me when they couldn't seem to get rid of bladder and kidney infections. Many found relief after cleansing the bowel and flushing the kidneys. Kidney failure is too prevalent in our society today for us to ignore it. Most of us know someone who knows someone who has or had this problem, so we should do what is necessary to protect ourselves and our loved ones from this disease. Let's begin to encourage one another to cleanse the kidneys annually. Annual cleansings of the kidneys at the beginning of winter safeguards us against kidney failure. However, if you have never cleaned your kidneys, today is the day to start. Call today for our cleansing formula to maintain and support the health of your kidneys.

THE POSITIVE SIDE EFFECTS
OF THE RAMADAN FAST

ALLAH REVEALED TO Prophet Muhammed (PBUH) that out of all the things He had given to the sons of Adam, the fast is for Him (Allah).

The beauty, serenity, happiness, and peace that accompanies the spiritual awakening one will experience during the blessed month of Ramadan is beyond one person's explanation. It is something one must experience for him- or herself to really understand. Abstaining from food, drink, and sex during the daylight hours, reading of the Holy Qur'an daily, and reciting extra prayers all become stimulants for this awakening process. Our Creator tells us in the Qur'an that He gave us the fast to teach us self-restraint. In addition, there are great health benefits (side effects) attached to the fast that are also blessings from the Lord.

As many people begin the fast, they will not sense a loss of strength at all. In fact, they will begin to feel stronger. Fasting is not an unusual experience. In the medical field, we observe that instead of losing strength while fasting, many gain strength. Invalids who were growing weaker on so-called healthy diets, which are commonly advised in hospital settings, will frequently begin to grow stronger as they start to fast. We sometimes see that the weakest person derives the greatest benefit from a period of abstinence. The weakness is not due to a lack of food, but in many cases, it's the result of a toxic state of the body.

Many think that the weak must build themselves up by eating. They are told they are too weak to fast. Even if the person is steadily growing weaker on what many believe to be nourishing food, the consumption must continue. In some cases, this is a great error.

Even when the patient is in bed and suffers from pain and fever, getting weaker each day because he or she is unable to digest food, many physicians believe we must keep feeding the individual. Many believe that if you feed the person in sufficient quantity, he or she will recover. Sometimes they will, but the feeding is not the cause of recovery. If the person dies at this critical time, overfeeding could be the cause of death. Will fasting save the person's life? Not always, but in many cases, the individual may have a better chance for recovery through fasting than eating.

Many believe that man is heavily dependent on food supplies and that if he misses a few meals, he will get weak and die. Healthy or sick, we are expected to eat three meals per day. We are supposed to ignore the distress signals of the body and continue to eat despite them. If there is no desire for food, eat anyway. If there is an acute repugnance for food, disregard it. If there is nausea, eat. If digestion is impaired and impossible, eat anyway. This is the popular misconception.

Thousands of people are fed to death annually in hospitals, nursing homes, and at home by well-meaning people who are ignorant of the regenerative properties of fasting.

In his book titled *Fasting Can Save Your Life*, Herbert M. Shelton points out, "In the animal world fasting is a tremendously important factor of existence. Animals fast not only when sick or wounded, but also during hibernation or aestivation (sleeping throughout the summer in tropical climates)." He also states, "Animals also survive forced fasts during periods of drought, snow, cold, and live for long periods when no food is available." Further, he says, "In mankind fasting has been practiced in various parts of the world over centuries for religious reasons, for self-discipline, for political purposes and as a means of restoring health. Only in recent centuries has the concept that he must eat to keep his strength has become a deeply entrenched idea."

One of the greatest side effects of the Ramadan fast is the detoxification process. Because of the body is not digesting food, it has more strength to cleanse and detoxify itself. The reality is that the more rest the internal organs get, the greater their ability to heal themselves.

The human body is designed upon the pattern of dynamism (fitra). Dynamic activity leads to dynamic rest, and dynamic rest leads to dynamic activity. For example, healthy children are in motion from the time they awake until the time they go to sleep. When they go to sleep, it's like they

ABDEL JALEEL NURIDDIN, ND, PHD

are in a coma. The more dynamic their activity, the deeper their sleep. The deeper they sleep, the more dynamic their activity. Our internal organs adhere to this same pattern. The more normal rest you give them, the stronger they become.

Fasting does not heal your body. The body is always in the process of healing itself if it has the strength. Fasting merely affords the condition the body needs for self-healing to take place. Fasting will not heal a broken bone or repair gum disease or get rid of tumors; however, the body has the potential to correct these problems naturally when the conditions are ripe for it, and fasting can assist.

Fasting will detoxify the bloodstream of impurities that circulate throughout the body, which ultimately causes the metabolic processes to enhance vital functions (sleeping adequately, thinking sharply, remembering, seeing, hearing, etc.). The body will optimize all these functions if we give it a chance. Fasting clears the way for the body to work on itself.

Weight loss is also a side effect of the Ramadan fast. Because most of us will be consuming fewer calories, we will mostly like reduce our weight. We are also cautioned not to be gluttonous when we break the fast each day. Clearing the complexion, sharpening concentration sharpened, and gaining more energy are all positive side effects of the Ramadan fast.

A nutritious Suhoor meal before daybreak will help direct the body toward cleansing and regeneration. A good vitamin and mineral supplement will help stimulate the immune system. A green drink will help in the detoxification process and assist in digestion.

Exercise some if possible, but you don't have to overdo it. The body wants the rest. You don't want to spend the entire fast sleeping either, but when you feel the need, rest. Keep the fast, read the Qur'an, and keep up prayer. And if it is Allah's will, you will have a great Ramadan.

ALLAH'S MERCY PERMITS US NOT
TO FAST IF WE ARE SICK

M ANY PEOPLE IN the past have questioned me about fasting when they are suffering from an illness such as diabetes. Some people need to eat and take medication to regulate their blood sugar levels. Allah will not hold you in violation of His injunction of fasting if you are sick. The rationale and logic of the deen (religion) are designed to benefit the person, not to harm the individual. The fast has been given to us for our benefit and not for the benefit of our Lord. If something that Allah has suggested we do threatens our lives, we are to use our best judgment regarding it. For those of you who may be diabetic or have some other disorder and fear displeasing your Lord by not fasting, Allah will be pleased with you if you use your common sense in this matter and preserve your health and possibly your life by not fasting.

If you are on medication and it is necessary for you to take that medication at regular intervals to keep your health, don't fear displeasing your Lord by not keeping the fast. Why would your Lord want to create illness in you by requiring you to fast? Our reason and logic tell us that this is not His intent. Thank Allah that He is merciful and forgiving. But even if one can't fast, one should desire to fast anyhow? Of course, you should want to, and Allah will bless you for the desire. And Allah says He will recognize your desire if you feed the indigent.

Let us be clear. These mitigating circumstances do not apply to someone with the sniffles or any other mild illness. For some, as you enter the fast and embark on the cleansing process, the body may suffer from cold or flu-like symptoms. Or you may experience mild skin eruptions (pimples), diarrhea, or what seems like an allergic reaction. These mild issues will soon pass, but if they seem like a hardship, then you will receive an additional blessing for keeping the fast.

Can one do a colon cleanse during the day of the fast? No! The fasting person may not consume food or liquid through any cavity of the body or intravenously during the daylight hours. One must do those practices before sunrise and after sunset. During the month of Ramadan, it could be a good idea to cleanse the colon through colemas or colonics. However, the body will be in a cleansing mode already, and you don't want to overdo it. Colon cleansing can be very tiring, and you don't want to give your body any reason to pull on you (the spirit) to break the fast. Fatigue has the potential to disturb your fasting spirit.

If one is in pain from a toothache or something else, can one break or not undertake the fast? Allah will judge us by our intent. Only you and your Lord will know how severe that pain is and whether it merits not fasting. Allah permits us to use our judgment, but Allah wants you to keep the fast.

Can a handicapped person fast? Yes, if they are not threatened biologically or psychologically by the fast, they are encouraged to fast like any other believer. It is the mind, not the body that needs self-restraint. Some handicapped persons are better suited to serve their Lord than those with all their limbs and mental faculties.

Is it permissible for the insane person to fast? To my knowledge, Allah has put little, if any, injunctions at all the insane. If we know certain people can temporarily lose their faculties if they don't take their medications, we must encourage them in a caring way to take their medication for their own sake and ours. If you think they understand, ask them to feed the indigent. If they don't understand, pray that Allah will have mercy on them because they can't follow the injunction. Allah wants us to love and care for one another and to be sincere advisers to one another in all affairs. All our actions are judged by intentions first.

The Sahur meal has been given to us as a mercy during the month of the fast. This meal, which we should eat each morning before the fast, is designed foremost to stop the fast from being a hardship on the practitioner, but it is also there to help preserve your health.

The person who has a need to take medication once per day, can take it in the morning with the Sahur meal; this gives one the opportunity to partake of the fast. Keeping enough nutrients in the system so that the blood sugar level won't fall too low and making sure there's enough water in the body to prevent dehydration are the benefits of the Sahur meal. Let us not underestimate Allah's wisdom by thinking He did not take these things into consideration. For health reasons, it is not wise to make a habit of skipping the Sahur meal. The Ramadan fast is designed to strengthen our lives in every way, especially our self-restraint.

Try to make sure you don't become constipated and dehydrated during the month of fasting. Drink plenty of water in the morning and after breaking the fast. You will probably modify the normal consumption of eight eight-ounce glasses of water per day. So drink as much water as you are comfortable with drinking, but try to drink more water than other liquids during the fast.

At a bare minimum, for the purpose of proper nutrition throughout the month of fasting, seek to start your day with water, something fresh, a fiber supplement, a good multivitamin, a multimineral, and if possible, a green drink.

For those of you who are sick, Allah has taken into consideration your sickness and has shown His mercy.

PREPARING FOR HAJJ

A NYONE WHO HAS traveled to Mecca and participated in the hajj will tell you that it is in your best interest to be in your best shape. While you will have the opportunity to leave home and experience sights that will boggle the imagination, this is not a leisurely vacation. The human spirit will be tested at times, and the strength of the physical body will be tested for endurance. Although the hajj won't commence until seventy days after Ramadan, early preparation is prudent.

It has been shown that most pilgrims have the mental toughness to endure the heat, the crowd of people, and other environmental circumstances, yet it's the strength of the body that makes the most difference. Approximately three million people all have their minds set on completing the same rituals at the same time, so the physical challenge can and will be confronting to your spirit.

Start a program for building health once you declare your intentions for hajj. It would be wise to start walking, jogging, or practicing some exercises you like doing with regularity to build up stamina and endurance. Drink plenty of water to support the immune system. Many people suffer from colds and flu-like symptoms while at hajj because they suffer from fatigue, stress, and lower resistance and also because people carry germs that can be transferred to others. If your bodies are not strong enough to endure the stress and the pace without losing their balance, you will experience the flow of mucus or undigested proteins. In most cases, this is needed, or the body would not go into the involuntary mode of cleansing. However, you can reduce some of its possibilities by subjecting yourself to voluntary cleansing and consuming nutrients in the preparation stage. Consume good nutrition to fortify the cells against the depletion of nutrients. The sun will pull fluids from your body, and electrolytes or minerals that supports your strength will be present in your sweat. By putting potassium, natural sodium, and complete proteins, such as brewer's yeast, bee pollen, wheat germ, spirulina, and grass juices, into your body in the preparation stage, you begin protecting it from depletion and imbalances while you are on hajj.

If you use my body chemistry support system on a daily basis during the preparation stage and exercise regularly, you will be in great shape for the hajj. Order your body chemistry support system today. It will help you get through life and the hajj with less stress and more endurance.

RETURNING HOME FROM HAJJ

THANKS ARE ALWAYS to Allah for the safe return of our brothers and sisters from hajj, and congratulation to the hajjis on their completion of this essential principle of their faith.

In the past, I have received many calls and comments from hajjis about the discomfort of colds or flu-like symptoms while on hajj and upon their return. The stress of the trip, the vitality of the sun, and the vitality from your enthusiasm all acted as healing factors in the detoxification of your body. To paraphrase our prophet Muhammed (PBUH), when you return from Hajj, you will be like a newborn.

The spirit of the newborn is clean, innocent, and full of vitality and enthusiasm. Your deep body tissue was laden with the toxic material you expelled before you left home, but the body didn't have the vitality to eliminate it. In addition, the stress of your travel and the possibility that you picked up a virus or bad bacteria acted as the trigger to release waste if your body culture was ripe for cleansing. However, the stress, the heat of the sun, and your enthusiasm were the primary factors of vitality started the flow of the mucus and undigested protein.

In "Preparing for Hajj," we talked about the necessity of building your body chemistry after Ramadan in order to make the hajj less traumatic for your body. Preparation is vital.

Now that you are home, continue to follow the body chemistry support system to cleanse the blood and the lymph system. Let the cleansing process run its course. If possible, don't use antibiotics. Make sure your bowels are moving three times per day, keep the friendly bacteria in your system, and use your digestive enzymes with each meal. The whole idea at this point is to keep the body in a reactive mode and not let toxic material settle again deep into the tissue where you previously removed it during the cold or flu you developed during the experience or after. Using bath salts once per week will reinforce the cleansing process.

FOUR ESSENTIAL STEPS TO BETTER HEALTH

Taking care of the nerves must be one of the most important things humans can do for better health. The nerves are the beginning and the end of your life. They are the first things that feed in the growing organism and the last things that feed in the dying organism. No one can be in his or her best health without periodically getting away from the regular routine and letting the nerves rest.

We should cultivate hobbies or pastimes that help us forget about the normal daily activities of our work that will give our nerves a chance to rest. The grinding pressure of a routine puts untold stress on the nervous system. Working our jobs without periods of vacation in different environments can be harmful to our health. We must allow the nervous system a chance to rejuvenate.

Regular domestic activities such as taking care of the children, husband, and the family produces stress on the nerves. Some people push themselves without breaks until they have nervous breakdowns. People must find something they enjoy doing that takes them away from the regular demands of everyday life. This gives our central nervous system a chance to rebuild itself and the autonomic nervous system a chance to adjust itself. It may be better for some to do it alone and for others with someone else. Your emotional behavior is a good indicator or gage for change. Making mistakes at a routine that you know you shouldn't be is a sign of fatigue. Letting little things that don't normally bother you start to irritate you is a sign of fatigue.

So too, the inability to sleep at night because the mind won't shut down is a sign of nervous tension and fatigue. These things and many others are telling you that it is time for a break. If you live in the city, a walk in the country may be just what you need. If you work with people every day and help them address problems, getting away from those problems and perhaps those people is necessary at times for the sake of your health. Taking a vacation with the family members and letting your guard down can be helpful. If your home life is stressful, you may need to get away from your spouse and the children and go somewhere alone to rejuvenate. This process will be different from one person to the next, and it depends on our personal needs. However, the most important thing is that you find something outside the normal routine that you like doing in order to give your nerves regular periods of rest. Try not to wait until you are at your wit's end before you recognize your need for a departure from the regular routine.

So too, make sure you keep the blood clean in the body. Make sure that your foods are as natural, pure, and whole as they can be. As a healthy person, you must scrutinize everything that you ingest. Sometimes we don't want to make our friends and relatives feel bad while they are visiting. For example, we may not normally eat what they have on their tables when we are invited to dinner at their places. In those cases, you may need to fast the next day to help clean up the blood from the previous day's meal.

Natural food or raw foods digest and are assimilated better by the body, and they help build and keep the blood clean. Try to stay away from herbicides, pesticides, colorings, fillers, and dyes in your food. A halal farm-grown chicken is a better (purer) source of food than a chicken that has never scratched the ground or seen the light of the sun because it was grown in a commercial coup. Deep ocean fish and farm-grown fish will be a better source of food than fish caught in our lakes and streams that are polluted with industrial waste. The purer the food, the better it will keep the blood clean.

It is better to eat wheat bread than white bread. White bread only uses a fraction of the whole food. Most of the nutrients have been milled out of the wheat to produce the white bread. Raw sugarcane is a whole food. White sugar uses a fraction of that food. Eating whole foods help to keep the blood clean and strong. Raw salt is a whole food, but white salt is another fraction of the whole. Try to eat your whole foods.

Circulation is also extremely important. Blood must circulate oxygen and other nutrients so that the cells can maintain good health. Exercise helps in the process of effective circulation. A fifteen-minute hot bath followed by a five-minute cold bath is very invigorating and promotes circulation in the body. Walking barefoot in the dew-covered grass is excellent for circulation. Walking barefoot on the seashore, first in the water and then on the warm sand, is good for circulation. The legs of the body are the pumps of the body. They facilitate the process of circulation more than anything else. Practice regular leg exercises to strengthen their ability to push blood to the brain. It's impossible for one to have very good health without proper circulation.

Rest is also important. Allowing yourself to rest is an indispensable element of better health. Too many people don't give themselves permission to rest. They become slaves to their professions. They work three or four jobs to try to get ahead, never thinking about their health. The stress of consistent activity without rest will undermine your immune system and ultimately produce sickness.

The vital organs of the body need rest to preserve their effective function. If you never rest them through fasting, they will become fatigued and shut down. Be mindful of these four essentials and practice them for better health.

EXERCISE: A GREAT TONIC FOR LIFE

N OW IS A good time to start your exercise program. Exercise is essential to the best health one can possibly obtain. Dr. Mick Hall stated, "If the benefits of exercise could be encapsulated, it would be the most widely prescribed drugs in history." The feeling of exhaustion as a result of exercise is a clear indicator of optimal health. Allah has truly blessed the human being with a body that can give the mind some peace and rest if we care for ourselves properly.

Movement is life. The more movement, the more life. Establishing a regular exercise program is one of the greatest personal investments of time one can make irrespective of age. Weight reduction, endurance, stamina, muscle toning, stretching, proper dieting, and the reduction of stress can all be a part of your program, and they all lead to great health.

The will to be your best at whatever you do should be a priority in your life. It's hard to believe that one can be their very best when the body is not in great shape. A weak body invites stress, fear, and mental weariness. Regular exercise will increase your energy by bringing into the body large amounts of oxygen. Consumption of large amounts of oxygen through exercise is the fastest way to build energy in the body, not to mention the least expensive. Some food and drink will give you energy, but it takes energy to burn it. We should not overlook the role of exercises in improving personal performance and overall health.

The mind works better when the body is toned. When the circulation of oxygen and bodily fluids are without obstructions in the body, we feel better mentally. Excretion, secretion, digestion, and elimination all function better when the body is exercised regularly. And because the mind and the body are so closely related to the proper function of the entire organism, it is almost impossible to separate the two. The health of the body will affect the mind, and the health of the mind will affect the body.

Exercise helps us be our best, and we cannot overlook our need for exercise. It takes enormous amounts of energy to raise up a community or build any enterprise. Exercise can save you from sickness and poor health. One of the best ways to use your time is practicing vigorous exercise. Exercise has always been good for healthy well-being.

INFANTS AND SOLID FOODS

D ESPITE WHAT A parent may think about a baby's body and its ability to digest and assimilate the same foods as an adult body, the reality is that it cannot process these things in most cases. Ignorance of the sensitivity a child's digestive system to certain food can lead to food allergies. Hay fever, ear infection, eczema, asthma, headaches, and arthritis in children can be traced to digestive problems stemming from the premature introduction of various foods into one's diet. In most cases, the best way to prevent allergies from developing in children is to introduce them to solid foods based while respecting the digestive system's ability to tolerate and digest them.

As we know, the Creator has placed milk in the mammary glands of the delivering female to feed the newborn child. The best nutrients the child needs for steady, healthy growth are present in the breast milk of the mother. The milk should be fed to the child up to approximately two years of age or the time of weaning. If you wean too soon or leave the child on the breast too long, you can harm the child chemically and socially.

Digestion in the body breaks down foods into simple sugars, amino acids, and fatty acids. Under the influence of digestion, these things become nonallergenic.

However, infants or babies are incapable of effectively completing this process until the age of seven months or so. The digestive system of the child must mature, and the more stable it is at the introduction of solid food, the better its ability to tolerate the food without allergic reaction. Babies sleep well when the digestive system is healthy. Some believe that solid food causes their babies to sleep, but that is a fallacy. The heavy food that will knock you out and leave you drugged when you awaken does the same to your child.

ABDEL JALEEL NURIDDIN, ND, PHD

Delaying the introduction of solid foods that instigate reactions in children is in the best interest of your child's health. The introduction of these foods should be delayed as long as possible. You can introduce foods into your child's diet in small amounts, and I would also recommend you only introduce one at a time. This will enable you to detect any reactions to that food. You should not give them new foods more than once in five days. During this process you should look for any change in the stool, behavior, or physiology (wheezing, sneezing, rashes, etc.). In the beginning, just give the child a bite, and if he or she doesn't experience a reaction, gradually increase the amount.

We must conduct additional research on scheduling the introduction of foods into diet. However, you may want to accept advice of naturopathic practitioners who have worked with children with allergies.

Carrots, poi, yams, squash, and zucchini are vegetables that children can generally tolerate. Beans, spinach, and peas should not be given before twelve months of age. Tomato and corn should be withheld until twenty-four months.

Raw fruit other than very ripe bananas should not be introduced before twelve months of age. Apples, peaches, and citrus fruits should be the very last fruits introduced. Many believe pears, plums, and apricots are the best tolerated.

Rice or oat cereal mixed with water or breast milk may be the best way to introduce grain to the infant at about nine months of age. Wheat, eggs, and cow's milk should not be given to an infant before twenty-one months of age, and you may want to refrain from giving cow's milk at all.

The following schedule includes more healthy foods and their approximate time of introduction:

- *Seven months*: hypoallergenic, pureed, mashed foods containing iron; 1–2 tablespoons per day, such as carrots, poi, squash, yams, broccoli, cauliflower, zucchini, Jerusalem artichoke, and sprouts (blended with water). Cook fruits, 2–3 times per day, kiwi, pears, prunes, cherries, banana, blackberries, grapes, applesauce.
- *Nine months*: foods high in zinc and good for the immune system, 2 to 4 times per day, sweet potato, cabbage, oatmeal, papaya,

potato, blueberries, lima beans, string beans, nectarine, peach, black strap molasses, split pea soup, millet, plum, rice cereal, beets.

- *Twelve months*: foods high in zinc and bulk; 4 to 6 times per day, corn squash, barley, chard, tofu, yogurt, parsnips, asparagus, avocado, egg yolk, rice, goat's milk, quinoa (grain), barley, buckwheat.
- *Eighteen months*: foods high in B vitamins and calcium, tahini, lamb, greens, kelp, eggplant, rye, beet greens, chicken, rutabaga, beans, fish, buckwheat, spinach, spelt, and teff (grains).
- *Twenty-one months*: foods high in protein, almond butter, egg, turkey walnuts, wheat, Cornish hen, cashew butter, pineapple, orange, and brewer's yeast.
- *Two to three years*: sunflower seeds, corn, peanut butter, clams, soy, cottage cheese, lentils, tomato, cheese, and beef.

ALLAH'S LAW WORKS THROUGH PROCESSES

F REQUENTLY, PEOPLE WILL ask me either by phone, during my seminars, or on my live television program what one can take for a particular ailment as if there is a single pill that will cure them.

The truth of the matter is that nothing from outside your body can heal you. And in most cases, it will take a combination of factors and processes for the body to heal itself. This is the instinctive wisdom of the body that Allah built into the cellular structure and encourages the body to heal itself. This healing mechanism needs encouragement through the uptake of nutrients within the body. The Creator is merciful. You only need to recognize this self-healing aspect of yourself and give it the proper raw materials or nutrients to work with, and instinctively, it will keep or rebuild your health. Ignoring this fact leads to complications in life.

I have found that sickness originates from a lifetime accumulation of toxic material in the tissue. Many people have never removed these toxins through intentional organ cleansing. People should thoroughly remove this waste from their bodies.

CELL DEGENERATION RETARDED
BY GOOD DIGESTION

FOOD CAN TASTE so good when we are eating it, even though sometimes we know we are going to pay a price later when it comes to digestion. However, there can be relief without pharmaceuticals.

Most people don't know that our bodies were not designed to do all the digesting of our foods. The foods we consume should assist in their own digestion. Then our bodies don't have to do all the work. All raw foods have predigestive enzymes in them. Nature put the enzymes into the food for digesting and decomposition in order to keep the ecological order in balance. However, the enzymes that are necessary for self-digestion of our foods are destroyed during the cooking process. Therefore, most people are using all their internal enzymes to digest their food, which takes away energy from other important functions of the body, such as healing, excretion, secretion, elimination, among others. Taking a digestion aid with our meals could preserve some use of our internal enzymes. There can be no life without enzymatic activity.

Every living thing needs enzymes to support its life. The human body is born with a bank of enzymes for metabolic and digestive purposes. Biologically, we are born with a limited amount of amylase to digest starch, a limited amount of protease to digest protein, and a limited amount of lipase to digest fats. Every time our bodies use some of these inborn enzymes, we deplete the bank. Most humans eat so much cooked food deficient of enzymes that in time their bodies don't have sufficient energy to digest their food. After that point, we cannot enjoy life without popping a pill to get rid of indigestion. Without digestive enzymes, gases develop, and acids are left unchecked in the gastrointestinal tract. This all leads to discomfort, inconvenience, and the degeneration of cell tissue.

There are thousands of processes in the body that are affected by enzymes. We can replenish our bodies by eating enzyme-rich foods or foods that still have live enzymes in them. Saliva does release the life force (enzymes) from the food after ingestion and mastication. Brewer's yeast, bee pollen, wheat germ, spirulina, and grass juices are complete proteins, loaded with life in the human body in their raw state. Foods will, in most cases, be better for our bodies in their raw state because they still have certain enzymes in them. However, because we eat so much cooked food, we should make a good habit of taking food enzymes with each meal to assist in the digestion of that meal. Then or bodies don't have to use all its enzymes to break down our food. This will retard the degeneration process and give us greater energy. Order my plant enzymes for better digestion today.

ASK FOR TESTIMONIALS IN BUYING NUTRITIONAL SUPPLEMENTS

S OME HAVE ASKED, "Out of all the nutritional supplements on the market, how do I know which ones are good?" The proof is in utilization. However, personal testimony from someone you know and/ or trust can offer an additional proof. Because the market of nutritional supplementation will carry with it mediocre and bogus products, caution and skepticism are understandable.

With an evolving industry of sales well into the hundreds of billions of dollars each year, there is bound to be rip-offs and scams in the industry. Your first criteria for selecting a good product should be personal testimony. What has that product done for someone else, preferably someone you know personally? Has the product previously addressed one of your concerns? Who is the manufacturer of the product? Is this company known for honesty and product integrity in the nutrition or health industry?

I also believe you should compare the price to quality. If you are going to pay top dollar for a product, it must be guaranteed to work.

In most cases, you will obtain your best products from an independent distributor. These products should not be found in retail outlets, and they will only be displayed in businesses where you must make appointments. The manufacturers of these products know they must produce a good product to protect their integrity and the integrity of their sales representatives. Conversely, retail outlets tend to depend upon previous advertisers and consumer knowledge, and they don't usually give a money-back guarantee.

Should I trust someone I know who's selling a nutritional product but who does not have previous academic or vocational education about nutrition? I don't believe Allah intended that we all have doctorates in order to help with our health or the health of others in a natural way. We are inundated today with preventive health care knowledge, and we should all be studying and sharing that information with others. However, you should question the salesperson about his or her personal use of the product, and you should also ask for documentation substantiating the efficacy of the product. If the person selling the product has not personally used the product line, then you should question your usage of that product.

Most products today in the preventive health care line are safe and don't have side effects. Reading your labels is also important. Remember quantity is not always the key to the better product. Our bodies work better on the quality of the substance ingested as opposed to the amount. Don't always look for the cheapest product and expect the best results. However, you can certainly find a good product at a reasonable price. Shop for quality and use your reason and intuition.

Look for quality products. You must also believe in a product for it to work effectively in your body. Again, your personal use and the personal testimony of someone you trust who has used the product line are great measures of value.

ADDRESSING HEPATITIS REQUIRES
A HEALTHY IMMUNE SYSTEM

H EPATITIS IS A viral infection that damages the liver. There are three types of hepatitis—A, B, and C. The method of contracting the virus can vary from bad drinking water to the use of tainted blood in transfusions to sexual transmission. In some cases, people fully recover, and in others illness is prolonged and results in death. Many people live with hepatitis without knowing they have it until they are tested or symptoms begin to show themselves. Symptoms include mild or severe fatigue, upper respiratory problems, nausea, vomiting, various joint aches or tenderness, muscle aches, headaches, loss of appetite, fever, jaundice, low blood sugar, anxiety, depression, nervousness, and visual changes.

Having a weakened liver can make one more susceptible to hepatitis. Toxic chemicals, alcohol, and drugs tend to cause liver cells to die. Medications that can damage the liver range from tranquilizers to chemotherapeutic agents, antibiotics, and anesthetics.

The gallbladder is seen by some naturopaths as the trash can for the liver. It must be flushed periodically of waste to help preserve the life of the liver.

Recovery from hepatitis largely depends upon restoring integrity to the liver. This can be done through liver cleansing with regularity and feeding the liver the nutrients it needs to maintain balance. There hasn't been much success with the use of interferon to destroy the virus. Consequently, allopathic medicine recommends a liver transplant. Today there are new drugs that will remove the virus from the body, and as a result, the body can make a full recovery. Ask your primary health care doctor.

One must recognize that the Creator gave us the immune system as the main defense of our lives. Its strength depends upon nutrients and sober habits of living. Too much of anything can disturb the balance in our bodies. However, the wrong things (e.g., smoking, drinking, drugging, etc.) will destroy it faster and more severely than anything, ultimately leading to degenerative conditions. Make sure you also avoid things such a bad coffee, white sugar, white flour products, saturated fats, bad hormones in red meat, and white table salt. These substances in extreme use are detrimental to overall health.

Not enough rest, a lack of water, unclean water, a lack of internal cleansing, and negative thoughts will affect our immune response. We need our immune system to protect our liver. If the immune system is healthy, it has the potential to produce its own natural interferon and other proteins that are designed to destroy viruses and other foreign nucleic acids.

If one is victimized by hepatitis, he or she should eat foods that detoxify and strengthen the liver. This includes alfalfa, wheat grass, barley green, among other plants, in addition to vitamins C, B, and E, selenium, and glutathione. There are many herbs that strengthen the liver too. Some of the most noteworthy are milk thistle and red clover. Because the immune system is such an integral part of this process, I suggest a strong immune booster such as a professional protocol of protease enzyme.

YOU DON'T HAVE TO COPE WITH YEAST
INFECTION OR CANDIDA ALBICANS

T HE ADVENT OF antibiotic along with the high intake of sugars have produced a modern-day plague that affects women, children, and men alike. Yeast infections or Candida albicans affect mainly women because yeast normally grows in warm, damp places, the vaginal tract making for an optimal environment. However, anyone can be the victim of these fungus. The symptomatic forms come in a wide variety and produce untold stress. But the good news is that by using a combination of diet and supplements, you can wipe out this menace. Those of you who have been victimized by Candida albicans can improve your health through nutrition and achieve higher levels of health by strengthening the immune response, and as a result, you will keep disease away from your health.

Human beings live in an ocean of bacteria that should be balanced in our bodies. Agents of infection (called microbes) travel throughout our bodies on a daily basis. Microbes can live in our throats, mouths, gums, noses, gastrointestinal tracts, and other places in the body. We should not fear these microorganisms (e.g., bacteria, viruses, fungi), but we must control them. They are a part of our human existence just as food and chemicals are. They are trying to eat us alive, and sometimes they succeed! Even if we die of natural causes, they will ultimately eat our biological remains. When our cells, tissues, and organs are healthy, we can effectively guard and defend against infectious microorganisms.

Host resistance is the factor that determines when and if the microbes will cause sickness or not. *Host resistance* is a technical term used by the medical industry to describe our body's ability to fight off infection. White blood cells (blood leukocytes) are a major part of the defense mechanism that destroys invading microorganisms that produce infection. Some of them ingest microbes and render them harmless. But for our body to manufacture the leukocytes, we must provide a major supply of amino acids, vitamins A, C, B1, B2, B6, and B12, biotin, niacinamide, pantothenic acid, and other nutrients. In addition, we need a balance of minerals and trace elements. Without all the amino acids, the production of white blood cells is greatly reduced, or manufacture may even cease. When this occurs, your host resistance is compromised, and then you develop a greater possibility or susceptibility to infections. This is based upon the law of cause and effect.

Host resistance also depends on the antibody system. When our bodies receive sufficient nutritional support, specialized protein substances known as antibodies are produced. These substances are made up of chains of amino acids (protein), and they attack invading microorganisms so that the leukocytes can destroy them.

Therefore, it is imperative that you understand the reality of illness. Infection does not take place because some *germ* decides it is going to attack your body. It happens because we have become nutritionally deficient and our bodies have become debilitated. This state gives the microbe the opportunity to set up residence. Simply put, an opportunistic microbe can only produce disease when the conditions are favorable.

Nutritional deficiencies seriously disrupt the integrity of the healthy immune response. There are also other factors in lowering of our resistance to infection, such as the consumption of large amounts of sugar (which paralyzes the phagocytes [eating] capacity of infectious microbes by our white blood cells), failing to get enough sleep, chronic constipation or diarrhea, anxiety, personal loss, too much physical stress, and more, but underlying all these are specific nutritional deficiencies.

Antibiotics are the modern-day treatment for bacterial infections, but they do nothing to address the deficiency of nutrition, which is the primary cause underlying the infection. In addition, antibiotics destroy the friendly bacteria in the gastrointestinal tract that are so necessary to keeping balance in the body. Antibiotics can produce fungal disorders themselves. While addressing one problem, they create side effects. Through repetitive use, they have been known to instigate yeast infections.

There are five major steps one should take to address yeast infections or candidiasis. First, you must destroy the yeast fungi. Second, you must eliminate all immune-suppressive drugs and antibiotics. You should only use these when it's absolutely necessary. Third, you must change your diet to starve the yeast of foods. Fourth, you must strengthen your immune system, which has likely become weak because of a lack of nutrients. Fifth, you must cleanse your colon to purify the bloodstream.

To eradicate a vaginal yeast infection, you can use KND-L, cajuput oil, lapacho, or white pond lily, which are all good herbal remedies. Accompanying the infection in some cases is a white vaginal discharge called leucorrhea. FEM-L, KND-L, and Usnea are herbal combinations produced by Pure Herbs Inc., and these compounds have shown themselves to be effective in eliminating the discharge. Remember that a woman's vagina cannot maintain a healthy state without the presence of lactobacillus acidophilus organisms. Additional symptoms include vulval, vaginal, and anal itching, sore throat with swollen lymph nodes, and tumors. Infants can develop colic, a sore tongue, food hypersensitivity, among other conditions.

Garlic, golden seal, mathake, whole-leaf aloe vera, peppermint leaf, and olive leaf are also used in the elimination of yeast infections. You must realize that the better the quality of the herb, the more effective it will be.

The need for a good multivitamin and a quality multimineral to strengthen your immune system is imperative.

Colon cleansing, liver cleansing, and parasite cleansing are all essential to good health. Stop using immune-suppressing drugs and consuming heavy sugars to live without yeast infections and candidiasis.

MAKE GOOD USE OF TIME WHILE YOU HAVE IT

S O OFTEN WE as human beings think we have time to wait. None of us know when death will come for us, but we know at some time it will indeed come. Because death is inevitable and we all know it, our tendency to put off what we know to be appropriate to preserve our health is irrational. It's easy to say at times, "We're all going to go at some point, so why care?"

While death is inevitable, it should not be our objective. Life is meant to be healthy, happy, and robust. The object of life is industry, growth, development, and prosperity. As humans, we should strive for joy, humor, and tranquility. We should look for a challenge to stimulate our minds and press on toward our goals. The meaning of life is enterprise, and advancement is its stabilizing force.

Too many Americans have taken a ho-hum attitude toward life, and now death has become a way out. As believers in a Creator, we should never take this attitude, which is a disease that leads to chronic physiological and social problems. The scripture tells us that after we finish one task, you should find another to give our energies to. We must always have goals that compel us to do something in the present. Keep pressure for improvement and advancement on yourself at all times. Stop to rest; however, don't stop too long, or else the bugs will destroy your garden.

We must make sleep a necessity, not an objective, or the roof may fall through.

I believe not getting out of ourselves what we know we should, somehow interferes with our self-esteem, and causes all types of problems of self confidence in our lives. The quest for progress should be present in the housewife as well as the businessman. This makes for a healthy society and a progressive future generation. Values are meant to be costly. Labor, effort, price, and promise are necessary to stimulate greater growth. We should all be willing to pay the price to receive the promise, and victory in every area of your life is the promise. Praise Allah for this day and your ability to see the sunrise and sunset. Thank Allah that you can breathe, eat, and sleep. Thank Him for the blessing of comprehension and judgment. Thank Him that you still have time to see your children walk, play, and grow. It is Allah who has blessed you with this day, and He wants you to make the best out of it.

Today is the day to make that difficult decision. Today is the day to start eating better. Today is the day to become more organized. Today is the day to finish your assignment. Today is the day to start your exercise program. Today is the day to apologize and ask for forgiveness. Not tomorrow but today.

WEIGHT REDUCTION AND THE NECESSITY
OF MENTAL REPROGRAMMING

S TATISTICS SAY THAT 65 to 80 percent of Americans are overweight. The medical industry is reporting that at least 20 percent of the population is on a diet, or at any given time, those people are looking for one diet that will help them lose weight. The good news is that you can lose weight safely and keep it off through neuro-associative programming, regulation of your eating habits, and exercise.

Many people reading this book who have sought weight reduction in the past will probably say, "I have tried everything I know, and I am still overweight." Well, if you are still interested in losing weight and protecting your health, I must encourage you to not give up and to try again. I believe those persons who remain overweight or gain additional weight are those who surrender to the challenge of weight reduction. They say to themselves, "I have tried. It's not going to happen for me. I can't afford to buy new clothes." Or they tell themselves similar statements to limit their beliefs about their potential.

Weight reduction and weight management must come from an empowering belief system. People must first believe they can before they will. I also believe you must have enough reasons to take the action that will lead to weight loss before you lose the weight sufficiently. You must desire a better physique, better health, a better career position, among other things, to motivate you to try. Without a reason to change, things remain the same.

You must consciously remember why you want to lose weight. The more pain you associate with keeping the weight, the more likely you will be moved to get rid of it.

Neurologically, human beings move toward pleasure and away from pain. Every decision that we make is associated with pain and pleasure. We seek to avoid anything that we see as painful to us. We are attracted to anything that we see a pleasurable. For example, eating chocolate or other sweets may be a pleasurable experience for you, but it may also cause you to gain weight, which is a negative experience for you. In order to break the habit of eating chocolate and sweets, you must associate pain with this activity. As long as eating chocolate and sweets are associated with pleasure, you will be motivated to eat them. However, if you associate pain when you think about chocolate and sweets, then the possibility of curtailing the activity becomes real. However, if you associate a bitter, foul taste or pain (weight gain) to these when you think about chocolate and sweets, you will be neurologically motivated to move away from consuming these items. This associative programming will work with any foods, attitude, or disposition.

Likewise, if one associates pleasure with drinking, dietary fiber, taking nutritional supplements, and exercise instead of pain (dislike of taste and inconvenience of taking pills), neurologically speaking, one will be motivated to utilize those products and stay active. Most people don't exercise because they associate pain with it. When you say that you don't have the time to exercise and yet remember that it will cause you to lose weight or stay in shape, you're actually saying that you do not want to inconvenience (pain) yourself. Or you are simply not willing to take time away from watching television, sleeping, shopping, cooking, reading, or eating (pleasure). There can be no result without activity, and all manifestation of desire must follow natural law.

In the present American environment, most people will not keep the weight off unless they learn how to eat, watch their diet, rest, cleanse, exercise, and keep this consciousness ever-present. This is biological law.

The desire to have a healthy physique is a natural one. However, to accept being out of shape, when what you want is a better physique, is a compromise of your better judgment. You should be working all the time to produce a better you because that is what Allah wants for you.

Along with neuro-associative programming, you do need good quality, effective nutritional supplements to assist in weight reduction. Don't be led into programs that tell you that you will lose thirty to fifty pounds safely in thirty days. For weight reduction to be safe, it must be a slow and gradual process.

Remember—in most cases, you will not lose significant weight without exercise. Regular walking at a brisk pace will do wonders for weight reduction. However, if you are not used to exercising, start slow at a pace that is comfortable for you and gradually build yourself up. For debilitated health problems, consult a health care professional. Joining a health spa and getting a coach has helped many people, and it may help you.

TONING THE BACK MUSCLES CAN
RESTORE PROPER ELIMINATION

T OO FEW PEOPLE today understand the importance of keeping the lower back muscles toned and their nerve flow adequate. Many people suffer from lower back pain and don't know the other factors associated with the condition. While the back pain grabs most of their attention, there are a number of other disorders that stem from the back condition that we should be aware of.

The central nervous system is centered in the spinal column. This column runs from the lower base of the brain down to the tailbone or coccyx. Proper nerve flow from the spine reaches every cell in the human body, and it keeps the electrical impulse steady to ensure proper metabolism. Without this nerve flow, tissue activity becomes sluggish or stagnant, which leads to localize constipation of glands and organs. This means elimination, secretions, excretions, digestion, and a host of additional metabolic process will not take place properly. This breakdown can lead to tumors, cysts, irritation, inflammation, ulceration, and ultimately cancer.

There are nerves in the lower back region of the spinal column that are attached to the transverse part of the colon. This portion of your colon runs across the stomach area of the upper torso, which includes the area from the waist up to the lower part of the neckline. The muscle action of the colon moves the feces through the transverse part of the colon from the right side of your body to the left side and out of the rectum. When the lower back muscles are not toned and the nerve flow is restricted in the lower back, a stricture can develop in the transverse part of the colon, which leads to constipation or a sluggish bowel movement. Colon problems are at the base of most all problems that occur in the body today. More fiber in our diets can eradicate many lower bowel problems. However, we cannot overlook the importance of the lower back muscles. They ensure proper nerve flow, which contributes immensely to proper elimination. Many are eating plenty of fiber, and yet their bowels are still sluggish. It is largely due to tissue congestion in the lower back muscles and/or structural misalignment.

I suggest people try a deep massage of the lower back muscles to rid the tissue of congestion, a chiropractic spinal adjustment in the upper part of the lumber region of the spine, and stretching exercises twice per day for the lower back. And using my body chemistry support system on a daily basis will help you tend to your gastrointestinal tract. In my workbook you can also find an entire chapter on back exercises that you can do each day that will restore the proper workings of the bowel.

KNOWING YOUR ACTUAL IDENTITY
IS RELATED TO HEALTH

MOST PEOPLE DON'T know how identity is actually related to overall health. When people think their minds and bodies are their only and true identities instead of tools that they use, then they can develop identity problems.

The true identity of the human being is spiritual. It involves the spirit or the soul of the person. The mind is a tool that the person uses to discriminate, judge, deliberate, rationalize, and reason with. The body is the physical form of human expression for you in the external or material world. While spirit, mind, and body all make up the entire organism, the most accurate description of this human *being* is spiritual. As humans, we say "I" to refer to our bodies and our minds. To say "my body" or "my mind" is to state that something else possesses or has authority over mind and body, which is true. The spirit should control the mind and the body. Maintaining the correct identity of ourselves and strengthening unity between spirit and mind is what brings happiness and health into our lives.

Loving, caring, and sharing are spiritual characteristics that emanate from the human being when there is unity between the soul and the mind of the person. When the mind is filled with greed, selfishness, envy, jealousy, and other negative traits, the mind and the soul lose their unity, and this disorientation leads to unhappiness. This unhappiness comprises servitude, grief, apathy, boredom, resignation, and the like in the life of the person. These states of consciousness translate themselves into sickness in the human body.

When we become ill with disease, we try to treat the body to satisfy the problem. Most people don't realize that the real problem is a lack of unity between their mind and their spirit first. It does not mean that we should not treat the body, but to neglect the disorientation between mind and spirit will only bring about a recurrence of the problem. The mind's irrational behavior, such as with selfishness or overindulgence, is not accepted by the soul or spirit without consequence. The spirit's vibrational response will be in disorder or disease within the body. The spirit will only accept what's good or useful from the mind. This leads to peace, happiness, and health in the body.

Proper relationships between parent and child as well as student and teacher are very critical to the health of the person. As parents, we procreate to perpetuate our species. However, the mind that comes into existence as a result of that process is here by the grace of Allah and *could* be of greater benefit to humanity than the parents' minds. We should not force our desire for the child on the child. That aggression might lead to disorders in the life of the child. The child's soul must find its happiness through its own conscience, or the child's mind may suffer disorientation. I know this is difficult to accept because we want the best for our children, but this is true. Our teachers in life are necessary, but they must not seek to override the conscience and intuition of the student. As parents and teachers, we must know where our jurisdiction stops. If the mind and the spirit are unified for good expression, then the Creator is leading that soul to a destiny of good. Our job can only be to direct the mind of the child or student toward the good that the infinite intelligence would have him or her express. The soul only accepts goodness, and it rebels against evil.

The beginning of all health, whether emotional, mental, or physical, rests in adopting a positive mental attitude and the proper identity of yourself. This will lead to harmony and unity between the mind and spirit. Prayer and meditation are for your soul, and the soul knows what and how much it is being fed. Keep harmony between your spirit and mind through accurate thinking, regular prayer, and meditation.

TAKE ACTION AGAINST HARMFUL PARASITES NOW!

THE NATURAL FOOD chain appears to be parasitic, but it's not. With parasitic activity, the parasite does not contribute to the survival of the host. One thing in nature is feeding off another for maintenance and survival purposes. Plants feed off minerals. Animals feed off plants and minerals, and man feeds off minerals, plants, and animals. And it appears that the earth feeds on man. This chain is a part of the natural cosmic order and must remain as such to keep its natural form. Should one form of life cease to feed upon another, this present order would cease to exist. So in the sense of survival, this behavior is very natural and necessary to preserve the earth's ecological order. Overpopulation by plants, animals, and man disturb this order.

At first glance, one could suppose that anything that is feeding on something else is a pest. Hyenas would be a pest for lions, and lions would be seen as a pest for the wildebeest. Whales would be seen as a pest for sea lions, and so on. And yet this is a natural behavior of organic life. However, when a parasite is feeding off a person, the organism disrupts his or her entire life and does not contribute to the host's survival. We must be aware of the parasites in the body because if we aren't, they will nest and colonize the gastrointestinal tract. The body can become a reservoir for parasites. They can thrive in the gastrointestinal tract, digestive tract, or any body cavity, organ, blood, tissue, or cell. Parasites, whether roundworms, pinworms, tapeworms, hookworms, protozoa, or intestinal flukes, all possess the potential to reside and reproduce while in a human host. These parasites can be transferred from contact with animals, contact with other humans, eating food, drinking water, using restrooms, and visiting other public places. Americans used to think that parasitic infections were only present in the Third World. However, today most Americans have parasites of some type. Many disorders (e.g., anemia, AIDS, and cancer) originated with parasites.

Parasites will nest in the lower part of the small intestine. This is where 70 to 80 percent of the food digestion takes place. These organisms are intelligent enough to eat the good nutrition and leave the host the remains, thereby creating nutritional deficiencies in the host. These nutritional deficiencies can lead to a lowered immune response or extreme fatigue syndrome. These animals must excrete waste after consumption, and this waste is very toxic to the human host. Many people who are suffering from anemia have hookworms on the colon walls, and these organisms feed on the host's iron intake. Children may have pinworms in their stool. Sometimes a parent can see these parasites outside the child's anal cavity where they come to lay eggs or die. The putrid matter that builds up on the wall of the large intestine is a breeding ground for parasites. This wall must be kept clean to preserve one's health. The parasite can often be seen in the stool of a host after colonics, enemas, or treatments with herbs treatments that are harmful to them. Today parasites are seen as more contributory to sickness than they were in the past. We must always fight parasites to remain in good health. Herbs such as wormwood, black walnut, and clove are known to rid the body of parasites. Every ninety days is a good interval for parasite removal. It is recommended that one goes through a five-day purge every ninety days, utilizing these cleansing herbs or others with the same effect to prevent parasitic infection. If you haven't used a formula to purge yourself of parasites, do it now.

STUDY TO UNDERSTAND FOOD AND
ITS PREPARATION BETTER

M OST PEOPLE DON'T have the faintest idea about food and its harmful and useful effects on the body, which is startling. Unfortunately, Americans are not taught about food at any level of education. For the most part, if you don't take courses that specialize in food knowledge, you will be virtually ignorant to food's value and proper utilization. Most people only know they are eating to prevent themselves from dying. They know from experience that if they don't eat regularly, they will become weak and fatigued. In addition, most people don't know anything about food groups, the proper combination of foods, the value of foods in their raw state, or how to eat to live.

I firmly believe that at one time in the history of human existence, it was best to eat all our food raw for their best nutritive value in the body. However, nowadays wheat, rye, barley, oats, beans, and nuts are very hard as opposed to the way they were in the beginning, when as scripture tells us food would grow year-round. Today there is a need for food to be canned, cooked, and baked. Yet I still believe in eating as much of your food in its raw state as possible. Your foods digest and are assimilated better throughout the body when they are eaten in their raw state.

Some of our foods today must be cooked because we cannot digest them when they reach you from the market. For example, if you eat your corn while it is green and its milk is fresh, it will be easily digested. But if you wait until it matures and gets dry, it will go into its starchy state, and the human body doesn't have the digestive fluid to break down raw starch. Therefore, in this state we need to grind and bake the corn, and if done properly, the starch again becomes grape sugar.

Too much protein in the diet can produce severe impurity in the system. In their milky state before they are fully grown, corn, wheat, peas, and beans contain only 4 to 5 percent protein, but they are very high in minerals and other tissue-building elements. However, when these foods mature, the protein content in wheat goes up to 8 to 14 percent, and beans can go up to 20 to 30 percent for protein. This undigested protein is what comes out in mucus form when one has a cold or the flu. This accumulation contributes to the toxic state in the body when it is not digested properly. Today it is almost imperative that we consume digestive enzymes to aid in the digestion of our meals, particularly the protein. We should try to eat all our beans, lentils, and corn in the early milky state when they don't have too much protein in them. Then it will be much easier for our bodies to handle them.

We must learn to cook our food in a way that will preserve its life-giving properties. If we destroy our good food in the preparation phase, over time our bodies will age faster than they have to. After you've eaten, your food is supposed to make blood. This can only happen if the life (enzymes) in the food isn't destroyed in the preparation stage. You should try to keep your food as simple and frugal as possible. Try not to cook more than will be eaten at that meal. Preparing and eating more than is necessary leads to acids, gases, fermentation, and spoiling of the food after it is eaten. Too much heat will destroy the enzymatic activity in the food and leave it lifeless. Eating your food in its natural state is always best.

Carrots, potatoes, tender beets, parsnips, cucumbers, and young turnips should not be peeled. The high mineral content is just beneath the skin. In cooking leafy vegetables, use only enough water to keep them from burning and never cook them longer than necessary. When cooking vegetables in water, always start with boiling water. Only use enough water to cook the vegetables. If any water remains, save it for soups and broth. That water will be heavy in its mineral content. However, the best way to cook vegetables is to bake them.

Fruits are very nourishing, and we should try to eat fresh fruit daily. It is a clean-burning food and is very cleansing to the system. If possible, stay away from cooked fruit. It will be very heavy in acid. Nuts and seeds should be consumed with a digestion aid because of their high protein content.

There is much to know about food to get the most out of your diet; however, if you don't seek to educate yourself in these matters, it won't get any better, and you won't see improvement in your health.

GIVE YOUR BRAIN NUTRIENTS FOR
PROPER PERFORMANCE

TODAY PEOPLE ARE beginning to realize that the brain must receive nutrients for its processes to work properly. We must remember things each and every day, and when we find that difficult, we question ourselves. We know that the data we are trying to remember is in the mind somewhere, but bringing it to the conscious mind is the issue. What causes us to forget? Without getting too technical on this subject, let's say it's a combination of stress, nutritional deficiency, and autointoxication. Simply put, this means one is not giving the brain the needed nutrients, not getting enough rest, and failing to cleanse the body's tissue adequately. Ultimately, the mind fails to open the files at the subconscious level for immediate use. The body is saturated with waste material that is impeding the access process. In addition, stress and tension restrict the natural flow of nerve energy.

At times when you stop trying the struggle to remember, the thought pops into your consciousness. The fact is that tension and stress cramp electrical flow. At the subatomic level of our biological makeup, we are comprised of electrical charges. This tells us that if we want our brains to work properly we must keep ourselves involved in stress-reducing exercises (e.g., regular prayer, meditation, plenty of rest, and physical exercise). Entertainment mixed with humor is one of the best tonics to release stress. And sometimes while we are engaged in relaxing entertainment, the mind will give us the answers we have been looking for.

Gingko biloba, an herb that humankind has been using for thousands of years, has risen in popularity as a remedy to improve brain function. It is a great herb for the memory and all mental processes. However, all herbs and nutrients will work better in our bodies if the cellular structure is clean. For the active ingredients in any herb to be used effectively, metabolism should have a clean surface.

As an example, if you have a furnace that burns coal and you don't clean the ashes out after burning the fuel, then the next time you use it, it will smoke and won't burn as efficiently. This will reduce the energy output of the engine and will slow the entire machine. However, if you clean out the ash, the fire will blaze with less smoke and give more energy to the machine. The cells in our brain and body work on the same principle. A faulty memory could be the result of accumulated ash, which in turn leads to poor metabolism.

The brain needs nutrient-rich blood and oxygen for its best performance. Create some exercise programs that will work your legs at least three times per week for twenty minutes each time. The legs are pumps that drive the blood to the brain. Tone the muscle in the legs, and you will see the mind become sharper. *Flabby legs lead to a flabby mind.* Lecithin is a great brain food. Use a tablespoon of my granulated lecithin each day. It will be great for your memory. For tissue cleansing, use my body chemistry support system, and keep up prayer and meditation to keep your stress level down.

LIFE CANNOT EXIST WITHOUT ENZYMES

Enzymes are catalysts or substances that speed up the rate of a chemical reaction without being permanently altered in the reaction. For example, hydrochloric acid catalyzes the hydrolysis (breakdown) of sucrose (sugar), and ptyalin, a salivary enzyme, catalyzes the hydrolysis of starch.

There is a need for enzymes to carry out every chemical reaction that takes place in the body. Every working organ in the body has enzymes to facilitate the life processes. Our vitamins and minerals could not be delivered to our vital organs without enzymes. There can be no digestion without enzymes. If we take in the proteins and we don't have the enzymes to digest them, they will putrefy in the body and become toxic. If we don't have the enzymes to digest carbohydrates, they will ferment in the body, and without enzymes, our fat consumption will become rancid as well. All this leads to organ and system imbalance, which ultimately causes disease.

As stated by Dr. DicQie Fuller, PhD, in her book *The Healing Powers of Enzymes*, body typing (biochemical individualism) is a unique way of helping clients keep and regain their health. While our bodies may have an enzyme bank, different body types can't digest certain food groups because of a deficiency of certain enzymes. If the body is deficient of protease, it can't break down protein. If it's deficient in lipase, it cannot break down fat. If it's deficient in amylase, it can't break down starch.

The endocrine system suffers from this lack of digestion process because of overstimulation. For example, people who crave carbohydrates and sugars stimulate *parathyroid* and *thyroid* activity until they cannot function properly. These people can't digest carbohydrates and starches effectively, so these foods ferment in the body, setting the stage for disorders such as fatigue, cold hands and feet, heart palpitations, nervousness, skin problems, weight loss, cramps in the legs, low blood pressure, obesity, insomnia, restlessness, lethargy, and other conditions.

People who crave fat can't digest lipids, and the lack of digestion overstimulates the *gonadal system* (sex glands). This body type produce disorder such as arthritis, gallbladder problems, prostate disorders, bladder situations, urinary situations, female problems, high cholesterol, allergies, psoriasis, and other conditions.

Then you have the body type that is stimulated by proteins but can't digest them. In this situation the *suprarenal glands* (adrenals) are abused and succumb to constant stress. Eventually, they may not function properly (a loss of adrenaline). These cravings and lack of digestion leads to disorders such as fatigue from stress, kidney conditions, body aches, high blood pressure, constipation, osteoporosis, gout, loss of hearing, insomnia, among others. Although you may be drawn to other foods, biochemical individualism (body typing) takes into consideration all of a person's unique qualities, including body shape.

There is also a body type whose *nerve/pituitary* system is overstimulated. These people suffer symptoms such as allergies, milk intolerance, skin conditions, aching knees, gas, fatigue, irritable bowel, anxiety, and nervousness.

Most people don't know that they have a genetic predisposition to intolerances or sensitivities to certain food groups. And yet each day they suffer the symptoms related to their body type. Finding out your body type and eating the foods that you can digest does much to improve your health. Consuming proteolytic enzymes, lipolytic enzymes, and polysaccharolytic enzymes to aid in the breakdown of protein, fats, and carbohydrates each day with and between meals will preserve your health in many ways. Each person is unique, and you should be conscious of what you are. Enzymes that come from plant sources, such as the ones used by the Genesis Health and Nutrition Center, become active as soon as they enter the body. Enzymes that are from an animal source are only active within the small intestine in neutral to alkaline pH.

ASSOCIATIONS BETWEEN MINERALS, EMOTIONS, AND OVERALL HEALTH

THE MIND AND body are so interconnected and interdependent that it is impossible to separate the two. Despite what most people think in terms of separation between the mind and body, every thought and emotion we think and feel has a direct effect on our cells and therefore our bodies. Allah says, "Man is created from the dust." The scripture uses the term *turab*, which not only means dust but also soil. Actual physical soil is much richer in mineral content than dust. These minerals include calcium, magnesium, sodium, potassium, phosphorus, to name a few. That's not that other minerals and trace elements, such as iron, copper, manganese, chromium, and zinc, are not important; however, the aforementioned are primary in energy production and oxidation rates (metabolism). The minerals in our bodies drive the endocrine, nervous, gastrointestinal, circulatory, and lymph systems. In addition, metabolic processes such as secretion, excretion, elimination, digestion, the production of hormones, and others are all dependent on minerals for adequate function. When our mineral levels are low or too high, the body loses its balance. If certain mineral ratios are out of balance in addition to the levels, then the body begins to suffer. Imbalance in the body can lead to emotional stress and psychological disorders. For example, if calcium levels are high, a person has a tendency to be stubborn, rigid, and defensive. If the levels are normal, the person is stable. If levels are low, the person is gullible, and his or her defenses are poor. If magnesium is high, a person has a tendency to be depressed. If normal, the person is flexible. If low, the person is weak. If sodium is high, the person tends to be volatile. If normal, the person is extroverted. If low, he or she is introverted. If potassium is high, the person tends to be an overachiever. If normal, the person finishes what he or she starts. If low, a person is depressed and indecisive. This mineral-emotional connection can also be seen with toxic metals, such as lead, mercury, and aluminum. If lead levels are high, it can lead to mental retardation and hyperactivity. If aluminum levels are high, it can lead to memory loss and dementia. When mercury levels are high, people can become nervous and psychotic.

It is of vital importance to know your mineral levels and address any imbalances to promote better health. For example, too high of a calcium-magnesium ratio (a.k.a. the blood sugar ratio) can lead to mental or emotional problems as well as diabetic conditions. A moderately high ratio can lead to hypoglycemia, and a low ratio can lead to dysinsulinism and other diabetic conditions.

Sodium and potassium (a.k.a. the life-death ratio) imbalances are associated with dysfunction in the heart, kidney, liver, and adrenal gland as well as immune deficiency. A high ratio leads to inflammations, adrenal imbalance, asthma, allergies, and kidney and liver problems. A moderately high ratio leads to inflammations. A low ratio leads to adrenal exhaustion. A moderately low ratio leads to kidney and liver dysfunction, allergies, arthritis, adrenal exhaustion, digestive problems, and HCL deficiency. A severely low ratio can lead to heart attack, cancer, arthritis, and kidney and liver disorders.

A calcium and potassium (a.k.a. the thyroid ratio) imbalance can lead to underactive thyroid, fatigue, dry skin, constipation, chills, lack of sweating, among other things.

A sodium and magnesium (a.k.a. the adrenal ratio) imbalance can lead to underactive adrenals, fatigue, depression, hypoglycemia, poor digestion, allergies, weight fluctuations, and burnout.

These are some of the most crucial ratios of minerals or electrolytes that must be balanced to ensure quality health. Most people don't know what their mineral levels are, which leaves them at a disadvantage when they are trying to improve or keep their present health. If you are already high in a mineral, you may not need more of it unless it is inaccessible to you, meaning that you have it in the body but cannot use it because of a health condition. If you are suffering any of the previously outlined symptoms, contact a health practitioner.

YOUR CHILD'S HEALTH IS IN YOUR HANDS

I REMEMBER A TIME some years ago when my daughter was in grammar school. One day after attending a program at my daughter's school for fifth-graders, the family stopped at a large grocery store to pick up a few items. My daughter and I went into the store alone while my wife sat in the car. Once inside, my daughter said to me, "Dad, I need something for my lunch."

I asked her, "What do you want to get?"

Her first response was cookies, to which I replied no! After that, I asked again, "What do you want?" Her second reply was again something loaded with sugar, and I was almost sure—Allah only knows—that had I asked a third time, I would have gotten a similar response. Although I was not upset, I began to question myself as a parent in regards to her eating habits. We left the store empty-handed with nothing for lunch. I thought, *If sugar is all you want for lunch, tomorrow will be a day of imposed fasting.*

The next morning before I left to drop my son off to catch his bus, I asked my wife what to get my daughter for her lunch. At her suggestion, I stopped at a twenty-four-hour grocery store to pick up a prepackaged lunch of processed turkey, cheese, and other things. While looking at the item, I knew it wasn't the best meal for my daughter's lunch, and my wife knew the same thing. Yet we needed something fit for consumption that wasn't too far away from her good nutritional habits, and we needed it right away. After I arrived home, my daughter thanked me for the lunch as she left. I said to her in an instructive way, "That is better than sugar."

She replied, "It has a Nestlé Crunch in it." I had overlooked that fact. With an innocent smile on her face, she also brought to my attention that the lunch had salt in it. Well, she had outdone me as a doctor and a parent.

I didn't say, "Give me that lunch." I accepted the reality that we had to better prepare her food when we could.

While my wife and I wanted the best for our family, as we all grew older, we realized that when it came to our diets, sometimes we had to compromise. We would try to make up for those compromises on the other end through cleansing and consistent nutritional supplementation. We wanted to raise our children with good eating habits that they would use later in life. Today, as we look back, we didn't do a bad job, but the situation is by no means perfect.

As parents, we must realize we are in a constant battle with the advertising industry about our children's diets. Therefore, we are fighting for our children's health. The rates of child illness because of colds, flu, dry coughs, scarlet fever, measles, ear infections, ringworms and other parasites, sore throats, and other ailments are all indicative of the battle we are waging for our health. We are fighting a foe that sometimes uses subliminal suggestions to influence our buying and eating habits. Yet through it all, we must be assertive and protect our family's health. You must act on what your best internal reasoning and instincts are telling you. You should not be motivated by outside voices. Our logic and reason must be under the influence of our natural spirit's rationale. We must protect our children and not leave them out for the wolves to gobble up. We are not to put our children at the end of the rank when it comes to prayer. Our children are to be in the middle of the ranks or between adults when possible. This should tell us the importance of our guardianship. Through some spiritual medium, Allah is always showing us the way we should live in this mundane world.

On a recent talk show, someone asked me what I thought about milk and red meat today. I responded by saying that the milk today did not resemble what it was like in the past. Much of it (though not all) has to do with federal regulations on homogenization and pasteurization. The FDA mandates that the milk go through these processes before it can be sold to the public. Both these processes destroy the enzymatic activity of the food, which is where the life of the milk is. Milk needs the enzymes lipase, protease, and amylase to break it down. These enzymes are naturally active in the milk before homogenization and pasteurization take place to help in the digestive process. However, heat destroys the enzymes. So here we have a food that Allah gave to us to provide a natural rich source of the mineral calcium and other wholesome nutrients, but because of processing, it is more harmful than useful with consistent use. The medical industry tells us that because of these processes, consumption will lead to allergies, ear infections, and respiratory problems, particularly in our children. If you want good milk for your child, you must find farmers who have cows that they use to provide milk to their own family. But I think goat's milk would be better for humans. It has less fat to break down, and the goats don't lick salt blocks as the cows do.

We have discovered similar findings for red meat. In its natural state, this meat is fit and lawful for our consumption based on the Qur'an. However, in most cases, because of people's greed, we are victimized and given poor quality food. Animals are fed steroids and hormones that are unnatural for human consumption. This is not a medicine to protect the animals from disease and safeguard our health. These steroids and hormones lead to bigger profits in poundage and faster time to slaughter, and that's why farmers use them. That's why the uproar against the red meat is so great today. It's not the meat. It's how meat is being handled.

Today it's against the law for athletes to use artificial steroids because it leads to unnatural performance. We shouldn't have steroids in our bodies either unless they are natural. The possibility of unnatural cell growth lies in the consumption of these artificial substances. We should also consider herbicides and pesticides when we eat red meat. I am not trying to discourage you from eating meat. I am merely pointing to things you should be aware of. Humans are omnivorous creatures. We are comfortable consuming both animals and plants, and we rule both kingdoms.

As you can see, our children won't be aware of these things unless we tell them. Surely there are things more dangerous than those that we and our children should be aware of, but these are important. Protect yourselves and your family's health before you reach the point where you have to say, "I wish I had done things differently." Your child's health is in your hands.

ACTION AND RESULTS ARE THE
NAME OF THE GAME

J UST HAVING KNOWLEDGE of health is not enough to bring about the results you are looking for. Knowing and doing are poles apart. The noted Harvard professor Dr. William James stated, "In admitting a new body of evidence, we instinctively seek to disturb as little as possible our pre-existing stock of ideas." Dr. James is implying that the mind does not want to shift or change its habits. While the conscious part of the mind will acknowledge the need for change, it is the subconscious part of the mind where the actual change of habit has to take place. It takes self-discipline to influence this pattern. We are creatures of habits—habits that can be changed because we are minds with bodies and not bodies with minds. The conscious mind is the only thing you have total control over. The subconscious mind becomes conditioned through habit and crystallizes into a certain form, which takes time to change even when there is desire, interest, and attention. Most people do not want to come out of the comfort zone of thought. They don't like how they feel or the results they are getting, but it is more comfortable to continue to think as they do than change their thought patterns and behavior. If you want to get the most out of what this book has to offer, you must be amenable to change. Ralph Waldo Emerson stated, "Do the thing and you will get the energy to do the thing." Faith and belief alone are not enough to bring about action. You must take initiative. Napoleon Hill stated, "Hope is the magic ingredient in motivation, but the secret to accomplishment is getting into action." If you are interested in building better health instead of simply fighting disease, you can do so through the knowledge and application of the principles in this book.

AFTERWORD

I WISH TO EXPRESS my appreciation for the consistent efforts of Dr. Abdel J. Nuriddin to keep our community informed of the latest advances in medicine. Too often our professional colleagues are not afforded the necessary time for journal review to keep up with the overwhelming explosion of knowledge in medicine.

It has been the traditional practice of Western medicine in the recent past that has held the conventional thinking that excluded the holistic approach to medicine, to the point of subtly suggesting that any other method of patient treatment borders on quackery. Recently, many patients with terminal diagnosis have sought the counsel and treatment outside the mode of conventional medicine with remarkable results. The best outcome for most of these patients has been the blending of the knowledge of not one but both worlds.

Dr. Nuriddin's research articles have rendered help not only to laypersons but to the professional health care provider, especially in terms of current theory, research, debate, and alternate treatment modalities. His writings appearing here in *Help Yourself to Ultimate Health: Know the Causes, Symptoms, and Solutions to Optimal Health* fulfill a need to reduce the dependency on commercial diuretics, antimicrobial agents, and psychoactive drugs, just to name a few, which too often render the patient with diminished mental acuity.

Of note in this book, wherein he recommended the specific seasons of the year as the appropriate time markers for cleansing the various major body organs. In all my ten years of medical school training and study that I was exposed to the optimal diurnal time for surgical procedures, still I was unfamiliar with the time for organ cleansing. Any viable organization to be secured in the present and guaranteed its place in the future must have continuing knowledge updates.

We wish to express our gratitude for Dr. Nuriddin's public, as well as private, support for many initiatives of Imam W. Deen Mohammed, whose works are strictly in the Qur'an and spirit of the Sunnah of Muhammed the Prophet (PBUH). Imam Mohammed stated, "The human mind is formed in the image and likeness of the knowledge that gives it birth; therefore, we need to be exposed to truth, because most of our physical complaints start in the mind." We should have our people become more conscious of their own personal, individual responsibility in caring for themselves. Caring about ourselves is not done just as an obligation that the self places upon the individual, but we do it as a way of thanking God.

We must see the whole person, not just the physical, biological person or the mental person, but we also must see the spiritual and the moral person. We must find a way to incorporate the language of moral consciousness, the language of human spirituality, into our effort to reach people—to make them more aware of their health and what they should do to stay in good health so that they're aware of themselves as total people and not just biological people. The best medicine is the natural matter from the material world (food for healing) that acts against a disturbance in the life of the person. Both the medicine and the germs are from the same one earth.

Prophet Muhammad (PBUH) said, "for every disease there is a cure."

Peace be upon you
Dr. Nasir Ahmad
Oral and Maxillofacial Surgeon

BACK-OF-BOOK INFORMATION

Website: www.drnuriddin.com

Email: genesishealthcenter@gmail.com

Office telephone: 336-852-3040

A HEALTH PROTOCOL

A protocol in this case is a method of addressing health disorders in a client's lifestyle. It comprises drinking healthy clean water, changing diet, resting, exercising, and applying nutritional supplementation in the consumption pattern. Also, in some cases, collaboration between the client's primary health care allopathic doctor and his or her naturopath doctor is required.

ITEMS FOR SALE

Book: *Help Yourself to Ultimate Health*: *Know the Causes, Symptoms, and Solutions to Optimal Health*

Workbook: *5 Principles of Balanced Health*

CD set: *Preventing the 8 Stages to Disease*

DVD set: *First 12 Lessons of the Master Key Series*

Water treatment systems: www.teamalkaviva.com/drnuriddin

TV show: Each Wednesday at 7:00 p.m.–8:00 p.m. EST on Cable 8 TV in Greensboro, North Carolina

Live stream: www.GCTV.VIEBIT.com

Blog talk radio: Each Monday at 8:00 p.m.–9:00 p.m. EST

Online at www.blogtalkradio.com/ghncenter

Dial-in number: 619-924-9881

Blog talk radio: Each Monday at 9:00 a.m. EST

Online at www.AM360.com

Dial-in number: 515-605-9891

Printed in the United States
By Bookmasters